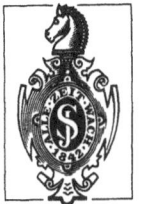

R. Texhammar   R. Schmoker

Stable Internal Fixation in Maxillofacial Bone Surgery

A Manual for Operating Room Personnel

Translated by T. Telger

With a Foreword by B. Spiessl

With 140 Figures

Springer-Verlag
Berlin Heidelberg New York Tokyo 1984

Rigmor Texhammar
Instructor
AO International
Balderstr. 30
3007 Berne, Switzerland

Roland R. Schmoker, M.D., D.M.D.
Department of Plastic and Reconstructive Surgery
Lindenhofspital
3012 Berne, Switzerland

Translator

Terry Telger
3054, Vaughn Avenue
Marina, CA 93933/USA

ISBN-13: 978-3-540-13593-7   e-ISBN-13: 978-3-642-69858-3
DOI: 10.1007/978-3-642-69858-3

Library of Congress Cataloging in Publication Data.
Texhammar, R. (Rigmor). Stable Internal Fixation in Maxillofacial Bone Surgery. Translation of:
Funktionsstabile maxillofaciale Osteosynthesen. Bibliography: p.   . Includes index. 1. Maxillo–Surgery. 2.
Facial bones–Surgery. 3. Internal Fixation in fractures. 4. Surgical instruments and apparatus. I. Schmoker,
R. R. (Roland R.), 1943–   . II. Title. [DNLM: 1. Facial Bones–surgery. 2. Fracture Fixation, Internal–instru-
mentation. 3. Maxillo–Surgery. 4. Surgery, Oral–instrumentation. WU 600 T355f] RD526.T4713
1984   617′.522   84-14040

2124/3130-543210

Foreword

Functionally stable internal fixation is of particular relevance to maxillofacial surgery, because it obviates the discomforts and inconveniences of intermaxillary fixation.

Given the biomechanics and biophysics of the skeletal system, the true immobilization of bone can be achieved only through highly technical means. Willenegger speaks of an "advanced school" of bone surgery which, when fully realized, will enable excellent results to be achieved even in the most difficult fractures. To accomplish this goal, ongoing refinements are needed in surgical methods and technology. Advancing the state of operative technique has been a central concern of the Association for the Study of Internal Fixation since its establishment 25 years ago. For this reason, a major priority of the AO/ASIF has been to develop its own surgical instrumentation.

With the help of technical commissions comprised of experts from medicine, research and manufacturing, the AO/ASIF has been able to develop and successfully test a line of surgical instruments whose trademark is known and respected the world over. For every specialty in traumatology and orthopaedics, including maxillofacial surgery, the AO/ASIF has developed both a basic and a special instrument set designed to meet specific anatomic requirements.

The present book is concerned with the maxillofacial instrumentation of the AO/ASIF. It is an excellent supplement to *AO/ASIF Instrumentation* by Séquin and Texhammar, also published by Springer Verlag. On the one hand, the book catalogues the various maxillofacial instruments and implants that are available, presenting guidelines on their preparation and usage. At the same time, it provides a deeper understanding of specific operative techniques and tactics. With its concise text and selected illustrations, it is a valuable reference not only for operating room personnel but also for the maxillofacial surgeon, in that it helps to standardize the "advanced school" of bone surgery. It is recommandable reading for the practitioner.

Basle, Summer 1984   B. Spiessl

Preface

Internal fixation of the jaws and facial bones is employed in trauma surgery, reconstructive surgery following tumor resections, and orthognathic maxillofacial surgery. It thus ranks among the most common operative procedures in this specialty.

The principles of the AO/ASIF (Association for the Study of Internal Fixation) were developed on the basic of systematic basis research, and their validity has been documented by an extensive body of data compiled by AO/ASIF groups in various countries (see Müller et al. 1977, Séquin and Texhammar 1981). This applies equally to the field of maxillofacial surgery (cf. Spiessl 1976).

The maxillofacial instrumentation of the AO/ASIF has earned an established place in the armamentarium of the maxillofacial surgeon. It is designed to provide a functionally stable internal fixation of the jaws and facial bones, and has found use in such areas as implantology and surgery of the temporomandibular joint.

The present manual was written for the purpose of familiarizing operating room personnel with the usage of the instruments and implants. The indications for and principles of operative procedures, and the preparation of the patient and instrumentation for traumatologic and corrective orthognathic maxillofacial surgery are discussed in a concise fashion. In addition, illustrations of table layouts and accompanying text provide a useful checklist for preoperative instrument setups.

We hope that this handbook will make the work of the operating room personnel easier. We hope, too, that it will stimulate active participation in these highly challenging operations.

We express our appreciation to Profs. W. Bandi, B. Spiessl and H. Tschopp, Dr. Dr. B. A. Rahn, and Mr. F. Séquin for their suggestions, advice and criticisms.

We extend special thanks to our secretary Miss M. Keller for her always prompt work, to our photographer Miss L. Schwendener, to our artist Mr. K. Oberli, to the operating-room and departmental nursing staff of the Inselspital Bern, and to Mrs. Bollier of the Outpatient Clinic of the Department of Plastic and Reconstructive Surgery of the University of Berne.

We thank the staff at Springer Verlag for their amiable cooperation and for their flawless work in bringing the book to press.

Berne, Summer 1984
R. Texhammar
R. Schmoker

Contents

1 General Guidelines for Maxillofacial Internal Fixation

1.1 Checklist of General Measures in the Management of Maxillofacial Trauma

1.1.1 Initial Management

Emergency Measures

- Maintain the *airway:*
  - Position patient on abdomen or side to prevent aspiration (caution: cervical fracture?).
  - In unconscious patients, the tongue may have to be pulled forward (e.g., with a towel clip) to prevent airway obstruction.
  - Look for loose teeth or fractured dentures (may require chest roentgenogram).

- Check *consciousness* and *pupillary reflex* (neurosurgical consultation may be advised).

- Control *bleeding:*
  - Anterior nasal pack.
  - Posterior nasal pack.
  - After intubation, packing of the oral cavity may be required; head bandage.
  - Further hemostasis is effected by maxillofacial surgeon.

- Check for *ocular injuries* (ophthalmologic consultation may be advised).

Clinical Examination

- *Inspection:*
  Swelling; hematoma; soft tissue injuries; asymmetric facial contours; enophthalmos; depression of the globe; telecanthus; "dishface"; unilateral or bilateral periorbital hematoma.

- *Palpation:*

  Tenderness; asymmetry; step; false motion; crepitus.

- *Function testing:*

  Sharpness of vision; double vision (with gaze straight ahead and at angles); ocular motility; sensation (trigeminal nerve); trismus; occlusion (subjective and objective); facial nerve branches; parotid duct.

Roentgenographic Examination

- *Semiaxial view of skull* and *jug-handle view.*

- *Orthopantomogram;* nuchodental contact view; isolated lateral view of mandible; bilateral Parma views of temporomandibular joints; occlusal view.

Diagnosis

- Fractures of the *condyle neck and zygoma* are most frequently overlooked.

- With a *lacerated and contused wound of the chin:*
  Examine wound area and contralateral condyle neck for fractures.

- With a *contusion in the buccal area:*
  Check for zygomatic fracture.

- With *mandibular fractures:*
  Check for contralateral condyle neck fracture.

Procedures

- In *edentulous* or *partially edentulous patients:*

  Where are the *dentures* or remnants thereof? (Important for exclusion of aspiration and helpful for later operative treatment; question paramedics, relatives or referring medical facility.)

- Every *mandibular fracture* in a *dentulous area* is treated as an *open fracture.* This will affect the timing of surgery and preoperative care (the oral cavity is sprayed thoroughly with antiseptic solution on admission and at intervals thereafter).

- *Le Fort fracture:*

  If general health is good, immediate surgery is indicated before the onset of swelling; otherwise surgery is deferred until neurologic status, respiration and circulation are stable, and facial swelling has subsided.

  Surgery is likewise postponed if *cerebrospinal fluid drainage* is suspected, in which case the monitoring of neurologic signs takes precedence. Confirm CSF drainage and its persistence; differentiate from nasal mucus or wound exudate. Nasal packing is avoided as it may cause retrograde flow and infection; exploration should be deferred until the facial bones have been stabilized.

  For *isolated nasal fractures,* reduction and fixation generally are deferred for 2–3 days until swelling has subsided.

- Facial fractures in patients with *multiple injuries:*

  The sequencing of priorities is done on an interdisciplinary basis under the direction of the emergency physician in charge, at which time it is decided whether facial injuries warrant primary or postprimary treatment. With *postprimary* treatment, main emphasis is on the control of bleeding, wound care, and other life-saving procedures on the neurocranium, chest, abdomen and blood vessels. Respiration, circulation and neurologic status are constantly monitored during this time. Afterward the patient is moved to ICU for further monitoring. Once respiration, circulation and neurologic signs have stabilized, CSF drainage has been confirmed or excluded, and facial swelling has subsided, definitive surgical treatment of the facial injuries is planned while concomitant injuries, such as limb fractures, are being treated. Usually this is done before extubation.

1.1.2 Preparation of the Patient on Admission

- Cold compresses; steroids if swelling is severe.

- Antibiotics as indicated (CSF drainage, fracture of dentulous jaw, contaminated wound, etc.).

- Meticulous oral hygiene with antiseptic solution spray.

1.1.3 Postoperative Care

- Reduction of swelling: – Cold, moist compresses.
- Oral hygiene: – After meals spray oral cavity thoroughly with antiseptic solution.
  - Start normal tooth brushing, followed by antiseptic rinse, as soon as possible.
  - Smear lips with Vaseline.
  - Air humidifier.

- Redon drainage: – Change bottles twice daily; suction the drains as needed to maintain patency; remove after 2–3 days.

- Mobilization: – According to surgeon's orders; will depend on patient's general condition (cerebral, pulmonary).

- Antibiotics: – As ordered.

- Check roentgenograms: – Before discharge.

- Hospitalization time: – 4–7 days for mandibular fractures.
  - About 1 week for midfacial fractures.
  - Longer for multiple injuries.

- Suture removal: – If healing is progressing well:
  - facial sutures are removed on 4th or 5th day;
  - neck sutures after 7–10 days;
  - intraoral mucosal sutures are removed after 2–3 weeks.

- Splint removal: – After 6–8 weeks.

- Cranio Fixateur externe: – Remains in place for 6–8 weeks.

- Follow-up examinations: – Schedule depends on associated injuries.

- Implant removal: – In 6 months to 1 year, often under local anesthesia.

1.2 Checklist of General Measures in Orthognathic Maxillofacial Surgery

1.2.1 Preoperative Planning and Treatment

- The foremost *indications* for orthognathic maxillofacial surgery are prognathism and retrognathism of the upper and lower jaw, open bite deformity, asymmetry of the mandible, and overbite deformity; the protrusion or retrusion of front teeth is a less common indication. Close teamwork between the orthodontist and surgeon is essential to an optimum result.

- Before corrective surgery is undertaken, an overall *treatment plan* should be formulated in consultation with the orthodontist. Growing patients usually benefit most from a combination of orthodontic and surgical treatment, while adults are generally treated surgically without orthodontic correction.

- When a combined surgical-orthodontic approach is elected, we favor several months of presurgical *orthodontic treatment* to bring the dental arches into a harmonious configuration. Only then do we begin actual surgical planning.

- The *planning of surgery* is guided by roentgenograms (teleroentgenograms, orthopantogram, dental films), photographs (frontal and profile views of face and teeth), and plaster models of the dental arches. An important part of planning is to *simulate* the operation on the plaster models. For corrective procedures within the dental arch, the models are sectioned at the proposed osteotomy site, and the fragments are placed in the desired position. The model is then used to construct a plastic plate which will serve as a template to ensure correct placement of the osteotomized fragments, and will also be wired into place along with the splint (likewise prepared beforehand). The actual repositioning of the jaw and subsequent functionally-stable internal fixation also require careful preoperative planning. This is done with the aid of *simulography,* which enables the proposed correction to be analyzed separately for each side of the jaw, and makes it possible to plan the line of osteotomy, the extent of the ostectomy, and the placement of lag screws.

- The *workup material* that will be taken into the operating room consists of the preoperative roentgenograms, photographs and simulographic record (Fig. 4), the original models and simulation models (placed on the table with the head light and dental drill directly behind the operator; see Fig. 1, p. 7 and Fig. 3, p. 8), and the acrylic template and splint prepared from the simulation models.

1.2.2 Preparation of the Patient on Admission

- Dental calculus is removed.
- Dental splints are applied.
- Individual teeth are ground as needed.
- Mouth is rinsed with antiseptic solution every 2 hours.

1.2.3 Postoperative Care

- Reduction of swelling: – Cold, moist compresses.

- Oral hygiene: – After meals spray oral cavity thoroughly with antiseptic solution.
    – Start normal tooth brushing, followed by antiseptic rinse, as soon as possible.
    – Smear lips with Vaseline.
    – Air humidifier.

- Mobilization: – As ordered.

- Antibiotics: – As ordered.

- Check roentgenograms: – Before discharge.

- Hospitalization time: – About 1 week.

- Suture removal: – If healing is progressing well:
        – facial sutures are removed on 4th or 5th day;
        – neck sutures after 7–10 days;
        – intraoral mucosal sutures are removed after 2–3 weeks.

- Cranial fixation: – Remains in place for 6–8 weeks.

- Follow-up examinations: – Every 1–2 weeks.

- Removal of screws: – After about 18 months.

1.3 General Preparations in the Operating Room

1.3.1 Recommended Locations of Personnel and Equipment

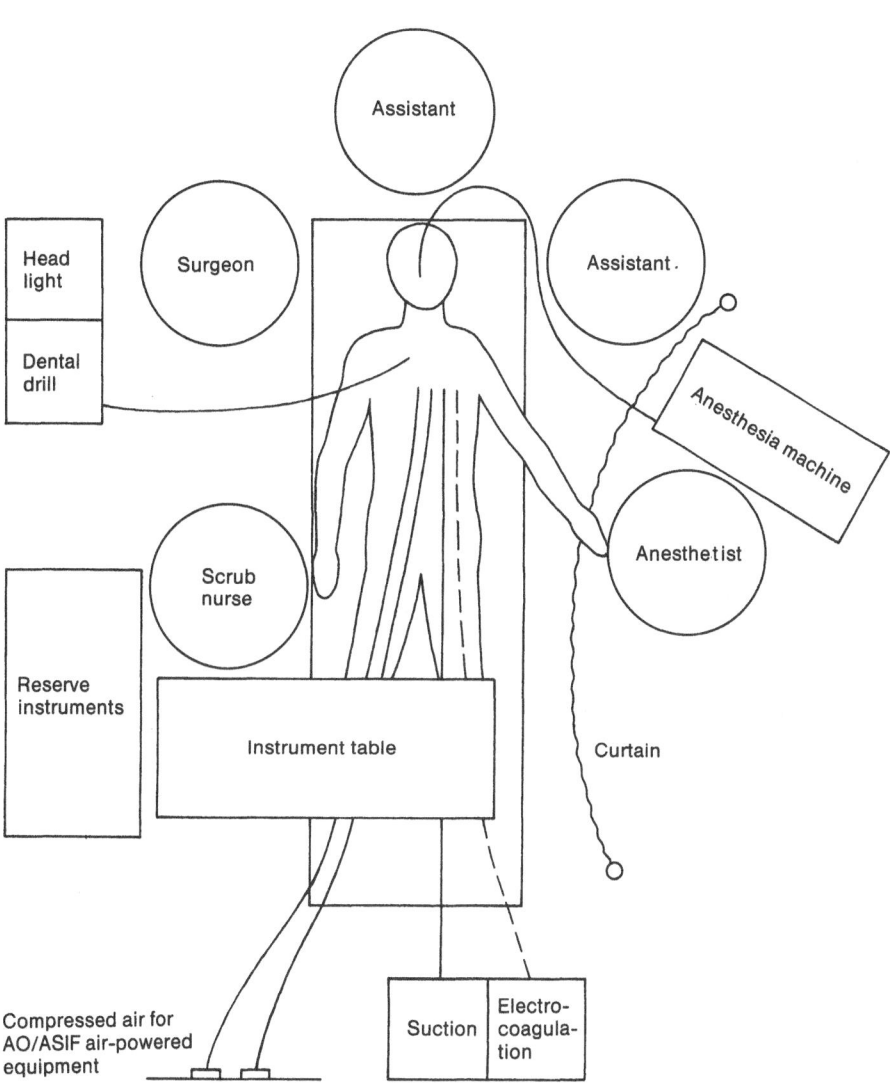

Fig. 1. Position of the surgical team and equipment for maxillofacial internal fixation

1.3.2 Preparation of Materials

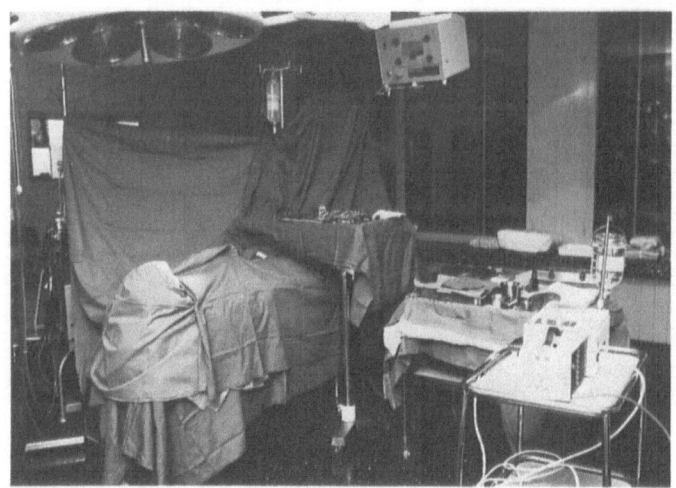

Fig. 2. Sterile draping of the patient, and placement of instrument tables and equipment for maxillofacial internal fixation

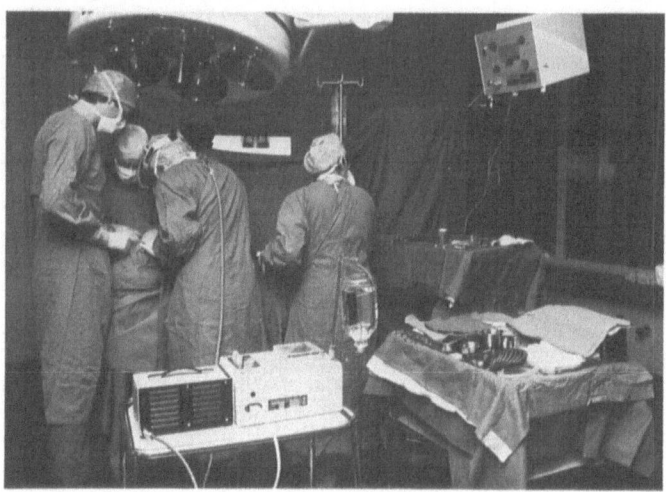

Fig. 3. Positions of the surgeon, assistants and scrub nurse for maxillofacial internal fixation

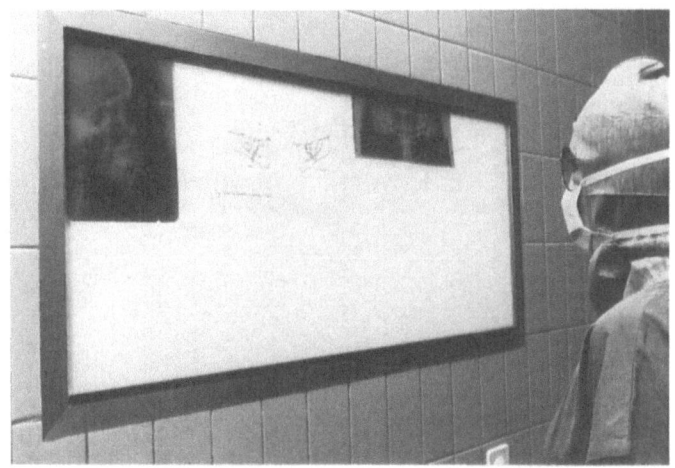

Fig. 4. Workup materials for orthognathic maxillofacial operations: teleroent-genogram of skull; simulography; orthopantogram

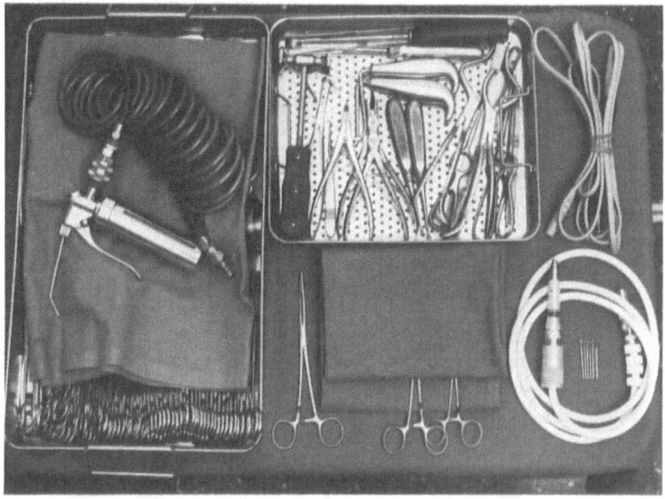

Fig. 5. Instrument trays for facial bone surgery

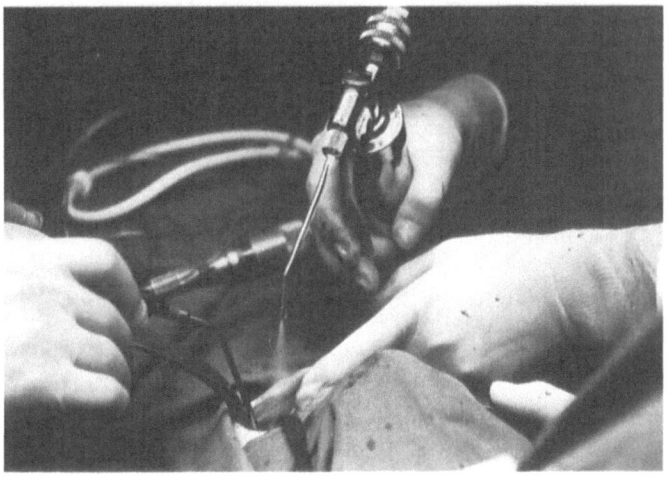

Fig. 6. Apparatus for intraoral spraying with antiseptic solution

1.4 Nomenclature

1.4.1 Anatomy of the Skull

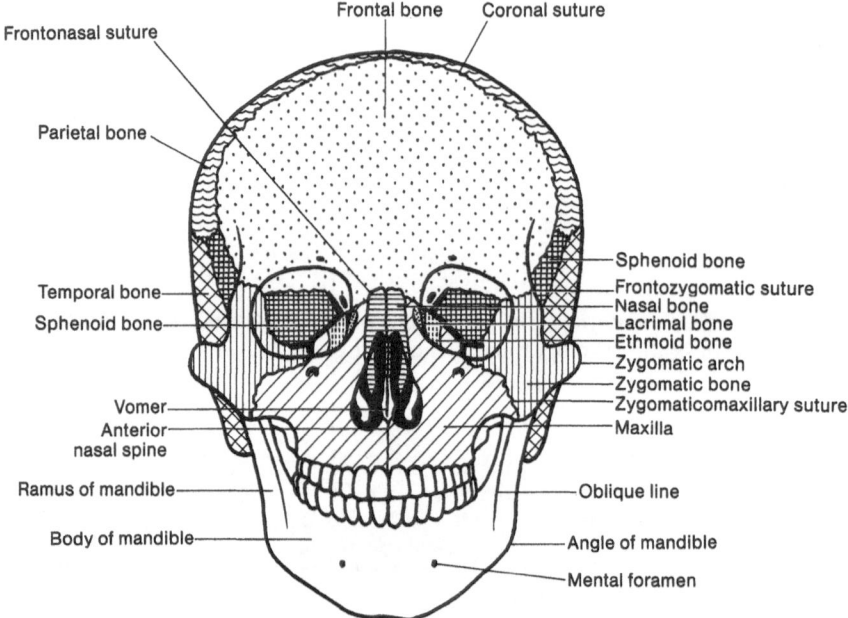

Fig. 7. The cranial bones, anterior view

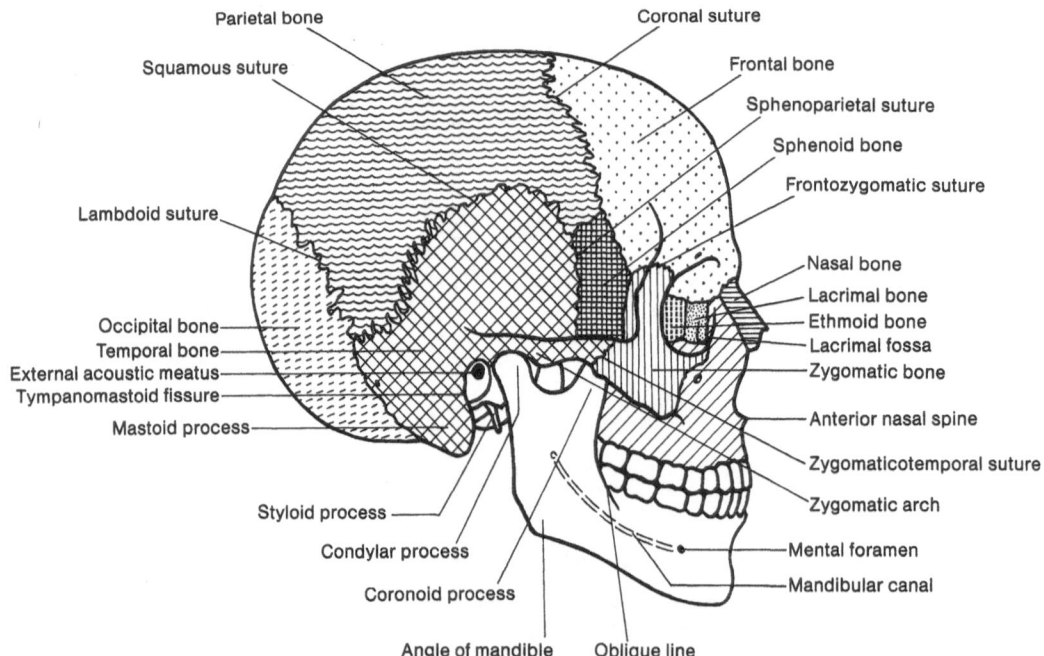

Fig. 8. The cranial bones, lateral view

1.4.2 Anatomy of the Mandible

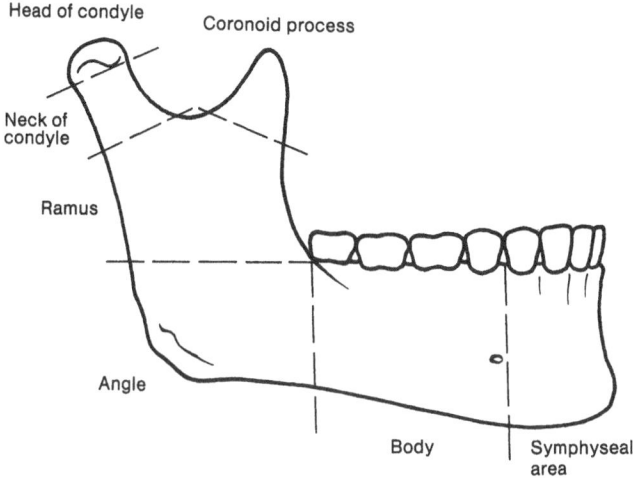

Fig. 9. Regions of the mandible

NERVUS TRIGEMINUS

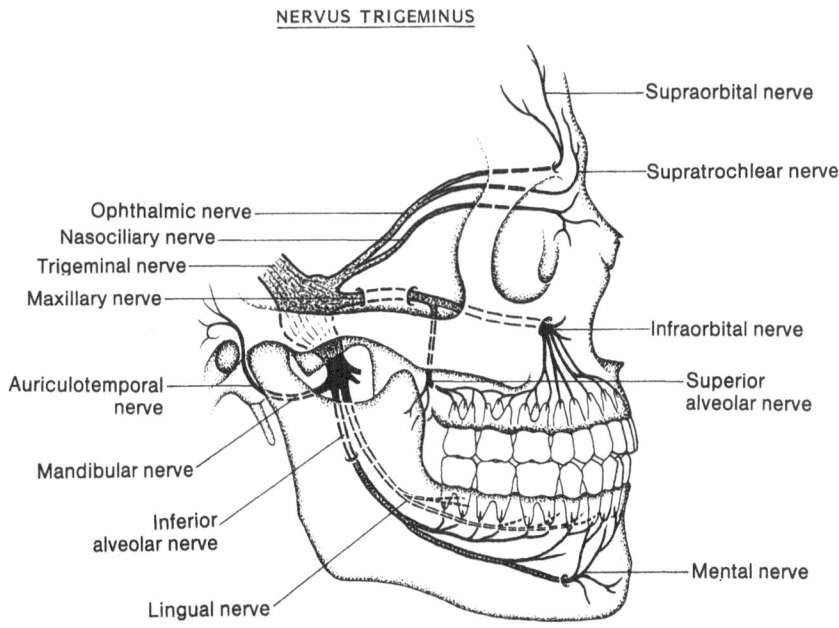

Fig. 10. The trigeminal nerve and its branches

1.4.3 Anatomy of the Dentition

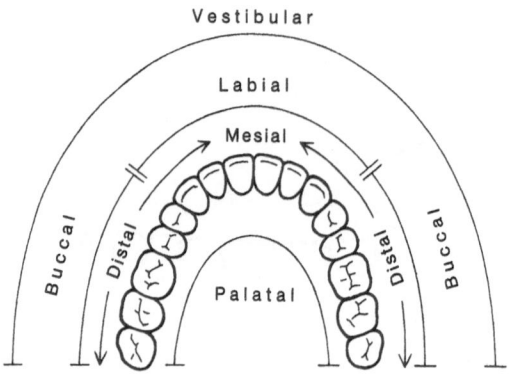

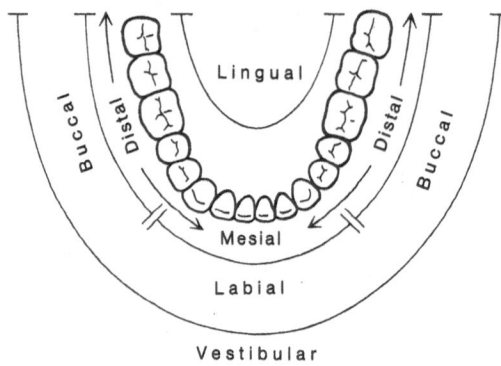

Fig. 11. Topography of the dentition

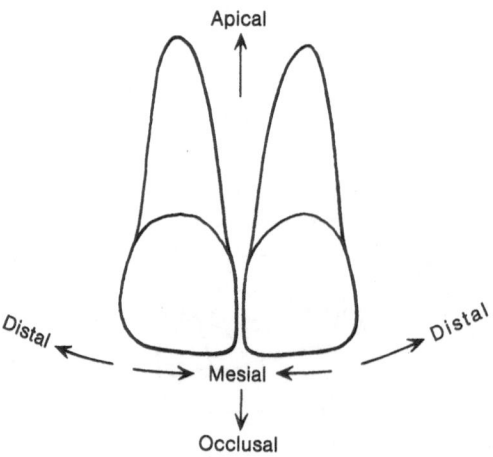

Fig. 12. Topography of the tooth

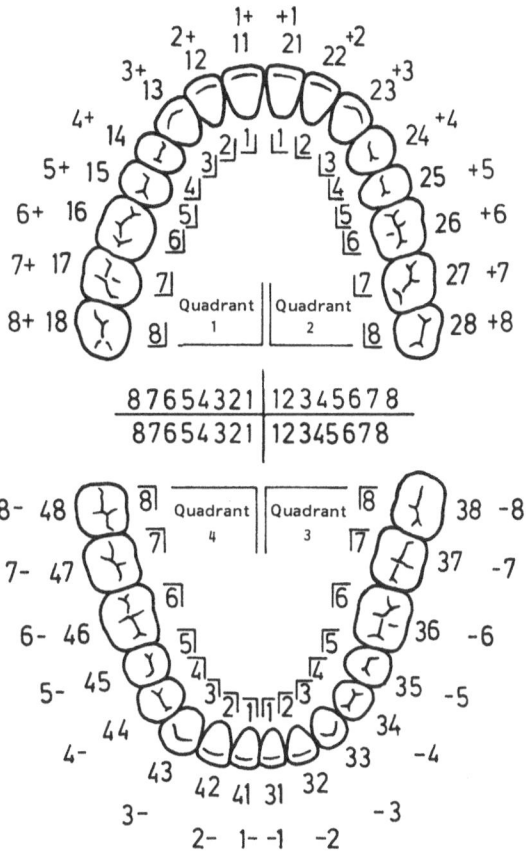

Fig. 13. Arrangement of the teeth and dental formulae

z.B. :

$$\frac{|2}{} = \underline{|2} = +2 = 22$$

$$\frac{}{3|} = \overline{3|} = 3- = 43$$

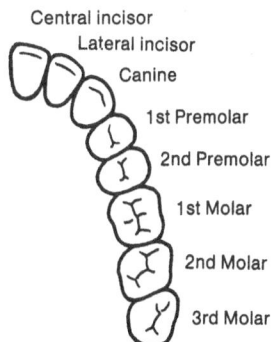

Central incisor
Lateral incisor
Canine
1st Premolar
2nd Premolar
1st Molar
2nd Molar
3rd Molar

Fig. 14. Nomenclature of the teeth

1.4.4 Various Drill Bits and Burrs

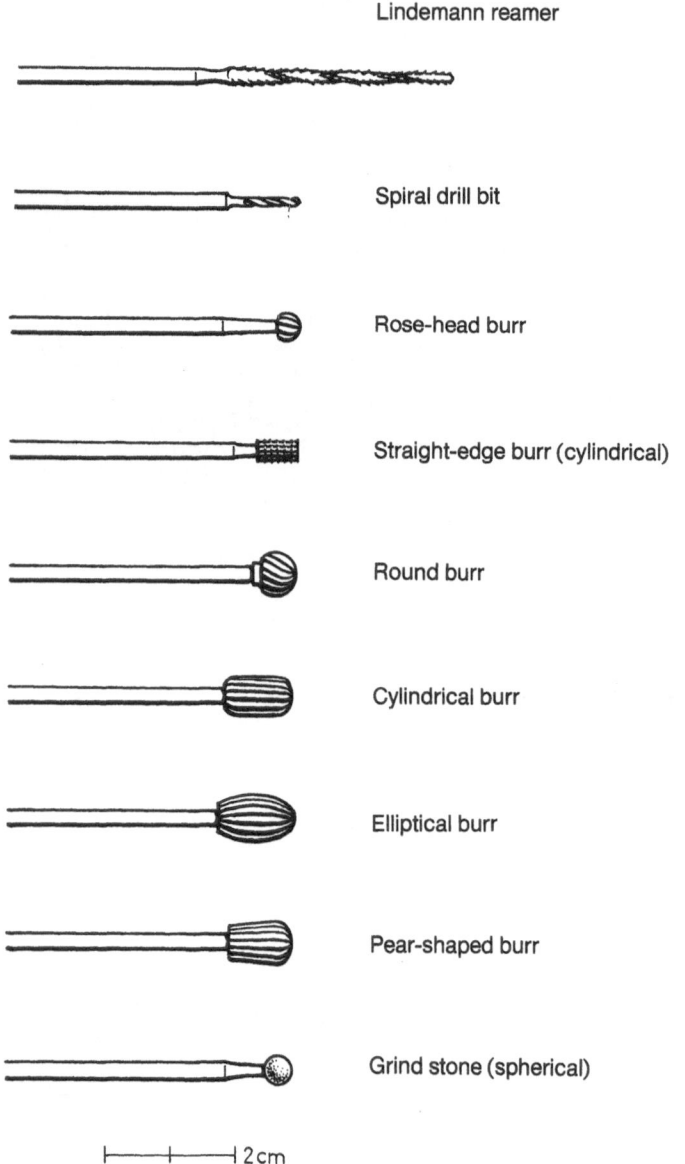

Lindemann reamer

Spiral drill bit

Rose-head burr

Straight-edge burr (cylindrical)

Round burr

Cylindrical burr

Elliptical burr

Pear-shaped burr

Grind stone (spherical)

⊢———⊣—⊣ 2 cm

Fig. 15. Drill bits and burrs for orthognathic maxillofacial surgery

2 Internal Fixation of the Mandible

2.1 Indications

Fractures of the mandible (except for condyle neck fractures).

2.2 Goals

Restoration of occlusion, accurate anatomic reduction, stable fixation of the fracture.

2.3 Timing

Definitive surgery may be primary (within 24 hours) or postprimary after vital functions have stabilized (circulation, respiration, CNS). In patients with multiple trauma, the fracture is treated concurrently with other injuries (with the possible exception of medullary nailing of the femur due to space limitations).

2.4 Diagnosis

- History
- Clinical findings
  - Inspection
  - Palpation
  - Function testing
- Roentgenograms

2.5 Preparation of the Patient on Admission

- Cold compresses; steroids if swelling is severe.

- Antibiotics for fractures of the dentulous mandible that are not absolutely fresh (every fracture in a tooth-bearing area is an open fracture).

- Meticulous oral hygiene with antiseptic spray.

2.6 Preoperative Preparation of the Patient

- Anesthesia:
  - Nasal intubation (tube may be sutured in place if required); line is passed over forehead to left arm.
  - Nasogastric tube.
  - Ophthalmic ointment.

- Positioning:
  - Head freely movable and accessible from both sides and from above (surgeon + two assistants).
  - Inflatable cushion under shoulders.

- Preparation of operative site:
  - Spray oral cavity with antiseptic solution.
  - For open fractures, wash with 1:1 solution of 3% H_2O_2 and physiologic NaCl.
  - Do skin disinfection of face and neck.
  - With closed mandibular fractures, sterile technique is not mandatory for interdental splinting (with open fractures splinting is done after the patient is draped). Repeat disinfection of oral cavity and skin.
  - Mark the border of the mandible, the fracture, the skin lines, and the proposed line of incision before draping.
  - Drape the patient as for thyroid surgery.

  Important: Internal fixation of the mandible requires the same asepsis as bone surgery!

2.7 Instruments and Equipment to be Prepared

- Instrument trays for facial bone surgery

- Splinting instruments

- AO/ASIF basic instrument set and implant set for maxillo-facial bone surgery (with special plates; DCP 2.7 mm, EDCP, 3-DBRP)[1]

- Dental drill

- Pressurized sprayer

- Head light for surgeon

- Suture materials:
  - Muscle: absorbable 4/0
  - Mucosa: nonabsorbable 4/0, braided
  - Skin: nonabsorbable 4/0, white intracutaneous
    nonabsorbable 5/0

2.8 Table Setups for Internal Fixation of the Mandible

- Instruments for splinting (see 2.8.1)

- Instruments for internal fixation of the mandible (two tables, see 2.8.2 and 2.8.3)

- If necessary, implants for mandibular reconstructions (see 2.8.4)

---

1 DCP   = Dynamic compression plate
  EDCP   = Eccentric dynamic compression plate
  3-DBRP = Three-dimensionally bendable reconstruction plate

2.8.1 Instruments for Splinting

Indications

- Preoperative interdental splinting and intermaxillary fixation (IMF) of mandibular fractures that are to be treated surgically.
- Splinting and IMF of condyle neck fractures that are to be treated conservatively.

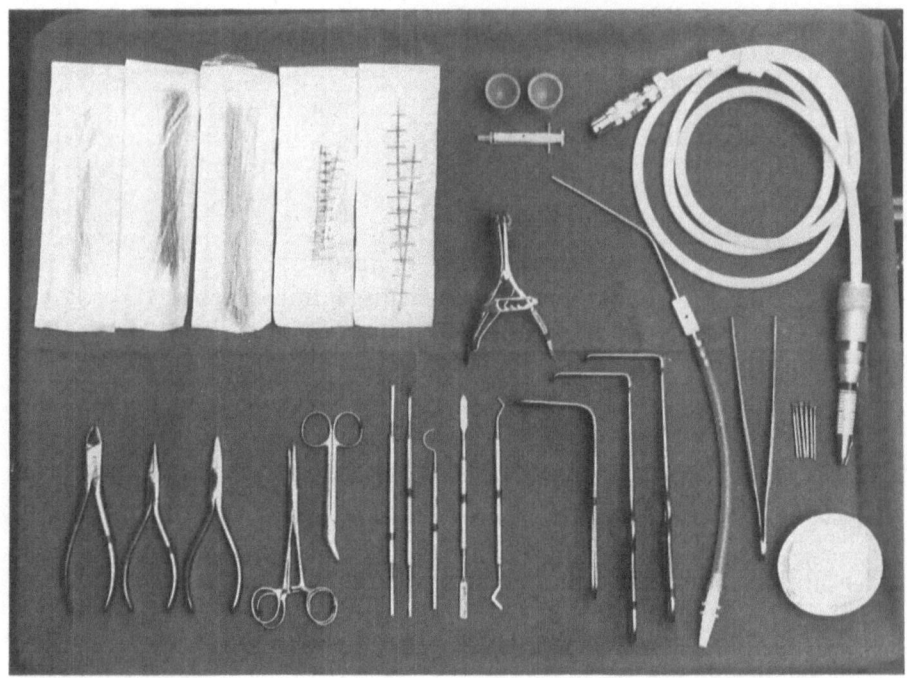

Fig. 16

Bottom (left to right):
1 Side-cutting forceps
1 Pointed forceps
1 Flat forceps
2 Bulldog forceps
1 Wire-cutting scissors, angled
1 Gauze packer, narrow
1 Gauze packer, broad
1 Dental probe
1 Cement spatula
1 Amalgam spatula
1 Tongue depressor
2 Langenbeck retractors
1 Fine suction tube with connecting
   tube
1 Tissue forceps
1 Basin with Vaseline strips
Connecting cable with micromotor,
handpiece, rose-head burrs and small
grindstone

Top (left to right):
Wires, 0.35 mm, 0.4 mm, 0.5 mm
4 Pediatric splints
2 Adult splints
1 Mouth gag
2 Rubber cups with acrylate
1 Syringe, 2 cm³

2.8.2 Instruments for Internal Fixation of the Mandible (1st Table)

Indications:

- Intraoperative splinting and IMF.
- Exposure of the mandibular fracture.

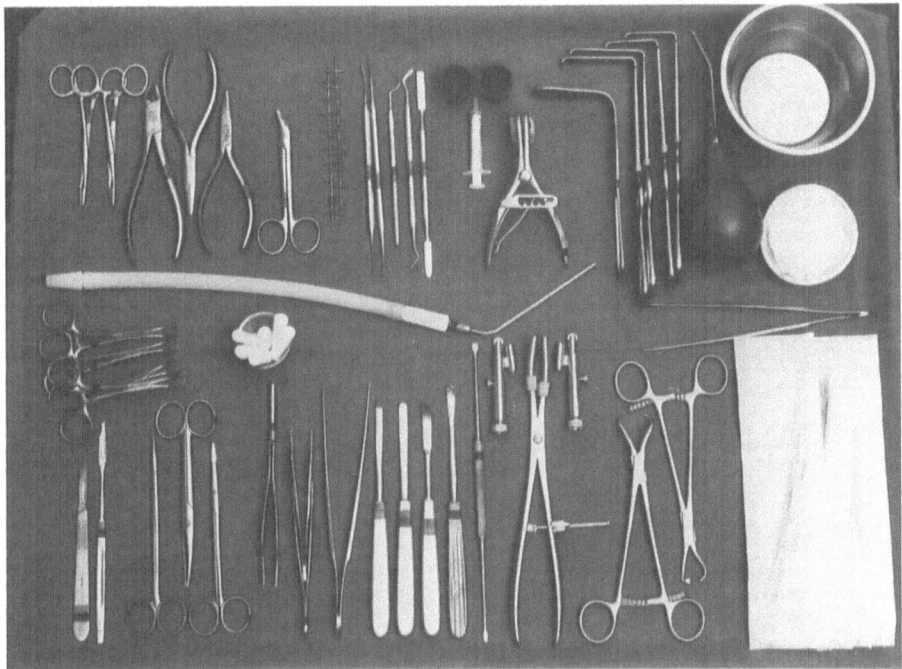

Fig. 17

Bottom (left to right):
2 Scalpels, nos. 10 and 15
2 Fine dissecting scissors
1 Mayo scissors
1 Coagulation forceps
2 Fine surgical forceps (extraoral)
1 Fine surgical forceps, long (intraoral)
3 Periosteal elevators
1 Periosteal elevator for protection during drilling
1 Fine periosteal elevator, long
1 Mandibular reduction forceps with 2 compression rolls
1 Reduction forceps with points
1 Holding forceps for small plates, extra-long
Wires, 0.35 mm, 0.4 mm, 0.5 mm

Middle (left to right):
4 Towel clamps
1 Basin with cotton rolls
1 Tissue forceps

1 Basin with Vaseline strips
1 Fine suction tube with adapter

Top (left to right):
2 Bulldog forceps
1 Side-cutting forceps
1 Flat forceps
1 Pointed forceps
1 Wire-cutting scissors, angled
2 Splints for interdental splinting
1 Gauze packer, narrow
1 Gauze packer, broad
1 Dental probe
1 Amalgam spatula
1 Cement spatula
2 Rubber cups for acrylate
1 Syringe, 2 cm^3
1 Mouth gag
1 Tongue depressor
4 Langenbeck retractors
1 Irrigating bulb
1 Basin for irrigating solution

19

2.8.3 Instruments for Internal Fixation of the Mandible (2nd Table)

Indications:

- Internal fixation of mandibular fractures (see Fig. 20).

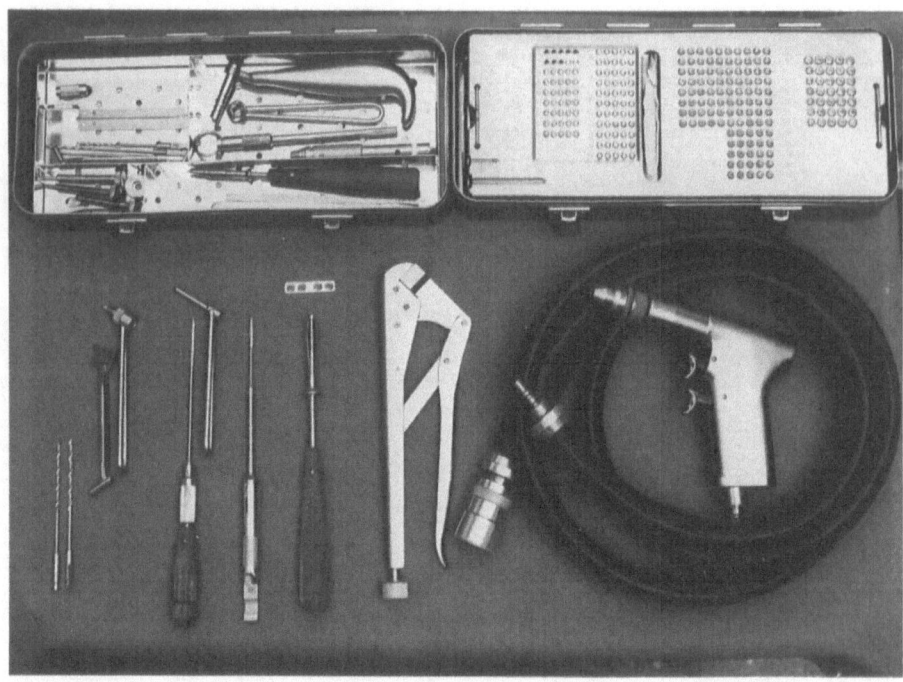

Fig. 18

Bottom (left to right):
Shown from the Basic Instrument Set
for Maxillofacial Bone Surgery:
1 Drill Bit, 2.0 mm
1 Drill Bit, 2.7 mm
1 Drill Guide and Drill Sleeve
1 Special DCP Drill Guide for Mandibular Plates
1 Tap, 2.7 mm
1 Handle with quick coupling
1 Tap Sleeve, 3.5 mm
1 Small Depth Gauge, extra-long
1 Small Screwdriver
1 Bending Pliers

Also:
1 Small Air Drill
1 Air Hose

Top (left to right):
Basic Instrument and Implant Sets for
Maxillofacial Bone Surgery
(shown: DCP, 2.7 mm)

2.8.4 Implants for Mandibular Reconstructions

Indications:

- Reduction and fixation of comminuted fractures, fractures with bone loss, and mandibular reconstructions following tumor resections.

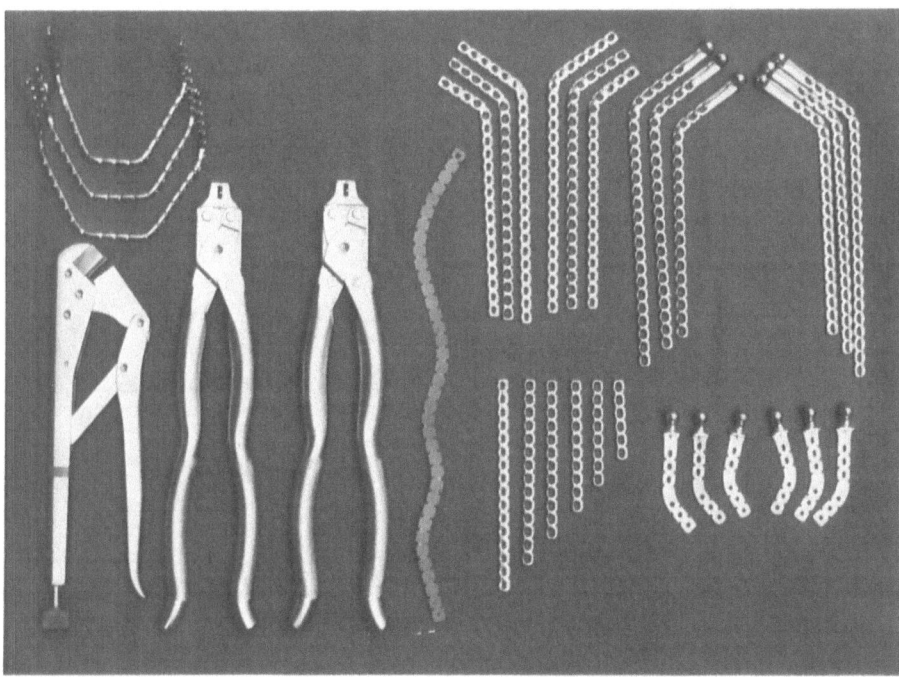

Fig. 19

Bottom (left to right):
1 Bending Pliers
2 Special Bending Pliers for Reconstruction Plates
1 Bending Template
Straight Narrow Reconstruction Plates
Condylar Prostheses, short

Top (left to right):
Mandibular Reconstruction Plates
– Bent Reconstruction Plates
– Bent Reconstruction Plates with Condylar Head

2.9 Examples of the Internal Fixation of Various Mandibular Fractures

Fractures of the Angle of the Mandible

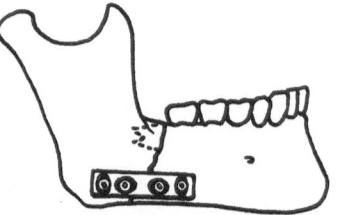 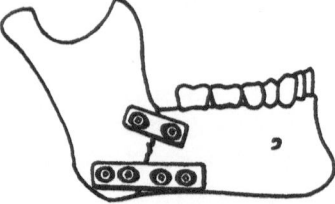

a Compression plating with an EDCP = Eccentric Dynamic Compression Peak (3rd molar prohibits tension-band plating)

b Compression and tension band plating with DCPs

Fractures of the Body of the Mandible

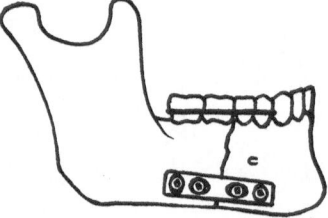 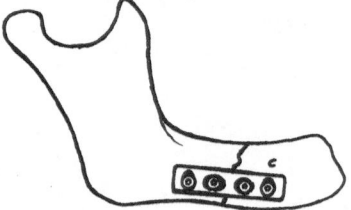

c, d Compression plating with an EDCP; a tension-band splint is also necessary in the dentulous jaw (**c**)

Fractures of the Symphyseal Area

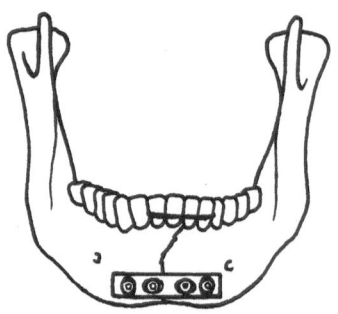 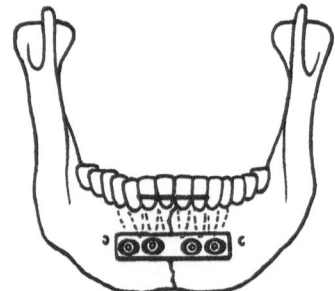

e Basal compression plating with an EDCP

f Infra apical compression plating with a DCP

Fig. 20a–f. Internal fixation of mandibular fractures occurring at various sites

2.10 Operative Procedure

- The pharynx is packed with Vaseline strips; the lips are smeared with Vaseline.

- Dental splints and IMF are applied intraorally.

- Further procedure:
  - Extraoral: the skin is incised and the platysma is divided.
  - Intraoral: the mucosa is incised.

- The fracture is exposed.

- The reduction-compression forceps is composed of the mandibular reduction forceps and the 2 compression rolls (see Fig. 21).

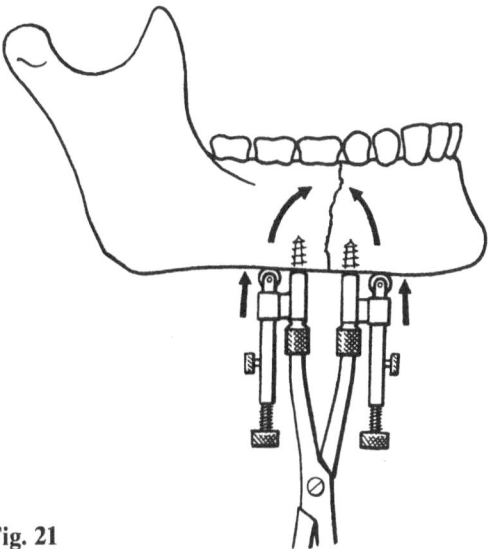

- With the 2.0 mm drill bit, one hole is drilled on each side of the fracture, keeping clear of the intended sites of insertion of the plate screws.
- The thread is cut (2.7 mm tap).
- The sleeves of the compression-rolls are attached to the bone with two cortex screws (2.7 mm, 6 or 8 mm long) and connected to the forceps.

Fig. 21

- First the fragments are distracted slightly to free incarcerated soft tissue. Then the fracture is reduced and compressed using the forceps handles and the two compression rolls.

- The bending template is used to determine the necessary plate length and contour.

- The plate is contoured on the template and then overbent slightly with the bending pliers.

- The first hole for the plate is drilled with the 2.0 mm drill bit and eccentric drill guide. If a lag screw is applied, the gliding hole in the near cortex is prepared with the 2.7 mm drill bit.

- The requisite screw length is measured.

- The thread is cut (2.7 mm tap).

- The first plate screw is loosely inserted, and the plate is adjusted so that the screw occupies an eccentric position away from the fracture line.

- The same procedure is followed in the other fragment.

- Both screws are tightened.

- When an EDCP is used: First screws are inserted into the longitudinal plate holes on either side of the fracture, and then into the transverse holes.

- The remaining screws are inserted into the longitudinal plate holes.

- The reduction forceps is removed.

- Redon drains are inserted.

- The oral cavity is sprayed with antiseptic solution.

- The wound is closed.
    - Muscle: absorbable 4/0
    - Mucosa: nonabsorbable 4/0, braided
    - Skin: nonabsorbable 4/0, white intracutaneous
                nonabsorbable 5/0

- IMF is removed.

- A spray dressing is applied to the wound, followed by adhesive strips.

2.11 Postoperative Care

- Reduction of swelling: — Cold, moist compresses.

- Oral hygiene: — After meals spray oral cavity thoroughly with antiseptic solution.
  - Start normal tooth brushing, followed by antiseptic rinse, as soon as possible.
  - Smear lips with Vaseline.

- Redon drainage: — Change bottles twice daily; suction the drains as needed to maintain patency; remove after 2–3 days.

- Mobilization: — Start on day of operation.

- Antibiotics: — As ordered; a 5-day regimen is customary.

- Check roentgenograms: — Before discharge.

- Hospitalization time: — 4–7 days for mandibular fractures.
  - Longer for multiple injuries.

- Suture removal: — If healing is progressing well:
  - facial sutures are removed on 4th or 5th day;
  - neck sutures after 7–10 days;
  - intraoral mucosal sutures are removed after 2–3 weeks.

- Splint removal: — After 6–8 weeks.

- Follow-up examinations: — At 1, 3, 6 and 12 months.

- Implant removal: — In 6 months to 1 year, often under local anesthesia.

3 Surgical Treatment of Midfacial Fractures

3.1 Indications

Fractures of the middle third of the face (see Fig. 22).

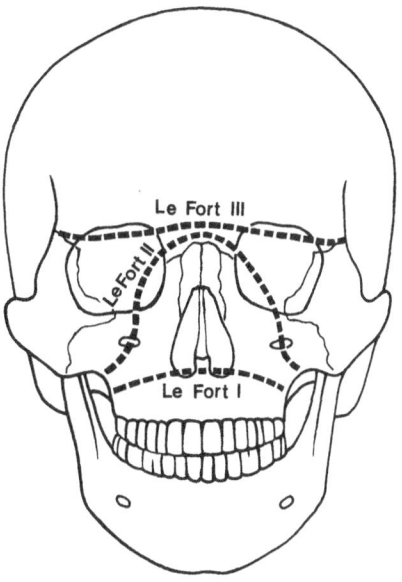

Classification

a) Central midfacial fractures
   - Nasal fractures
   - Le Fort I
   - Le Fort II
   - Le Fort III

b) Lateral midfacial fractures
   - Fractures of the zygoma
   - Fractures of the zygomatic arch
   - Orbital blow-out fractures

Fig. 22

3.2 Goals

Restoration of occlusion, accurate anatomic reduction, stable fixation of the fracture.

3.3 Timing

Definitive surgery may be primary (within 24 hours) or postprimary after vital functions have stabilized (circulation, respiration, CNS). In patients with multiple trauma, the fracture is treated concurrently with other injuries (with the possible exception of medullary nailing of the femur due to space limitations). With heavy bleeding from the maxillary artery, packing of the maxillary sinus may afford adequate hemostasis. Postprimary surgery is also indicated if swelling is severe.

3.4 Diagnosis

- History
- Clinical findings
  - Inspection
  - Palpation
  - Function testing
  - Examination for CSF drainage
- Roentgenograms

3.5 Preparation of the Patient on Admission

- Cold compresses; steroids if swelling is severe.
- Meticulous oral hygiene with antiseptic solution spray.

3.6 Preoperative Preparation of the Patient

- Anesthesia: – Nasal intubation with line passed over forehead to left arm (for splinting and IMF); afterward line is passed over chin to left arm (for midfacial access).

- Positioning: – Head freely movable and accessible from both sides and from above (surgeon + two assistants).
  - Inflatable cushion under shoulders.

- Preparation of operative site:
  - Spray oral cavity with antiseptic solution.
  - For open fractures, wash with 1 : 1 solution of 3% H_2O_2 and physiologic NaCl.
  - Do skin disinfection of face and neck.
  - With closed midfacial fractures, sterile technique is not mandatory for interdental splinting (with open fractures splinting is done after the patient is draped). Repeat disinfection of oral cavity and skin.
  - Drape the patient as for thyroid surgery, with the eyes draped free.

3.7 Instruments and Equipment to be Prepared

- Instrument trays for facial bone surgery
- Splinting instruments
- AO/ASIF Basic Instrument Set and Implant Set for Maxillofacial Bone Surgery (mini-implants) are needed in special cases
- Cranio Fixateur externe
- Dental drill
- Pressurized sprayer
- Head light for surgeon
- Suture materials:
  - Muscle: absorbable 5/0
  - Mucosa: nonabsorbable 4/0, braided
  - Skin: nonabsorbable 5/0

3.8 Table Setups for Midfacial Fractures

- Instruments for splinting (see 3.8.1)
- Instruments for internal fixation of the maxilla (see 3.8.2)
- Instruments for internal fixation of the orbit (see 3.8.3)
- Cranio Fixateur externe (see 3.8.4)

3.8.1 Instruments for Splinting

Indications:

- Le Fort fractures.

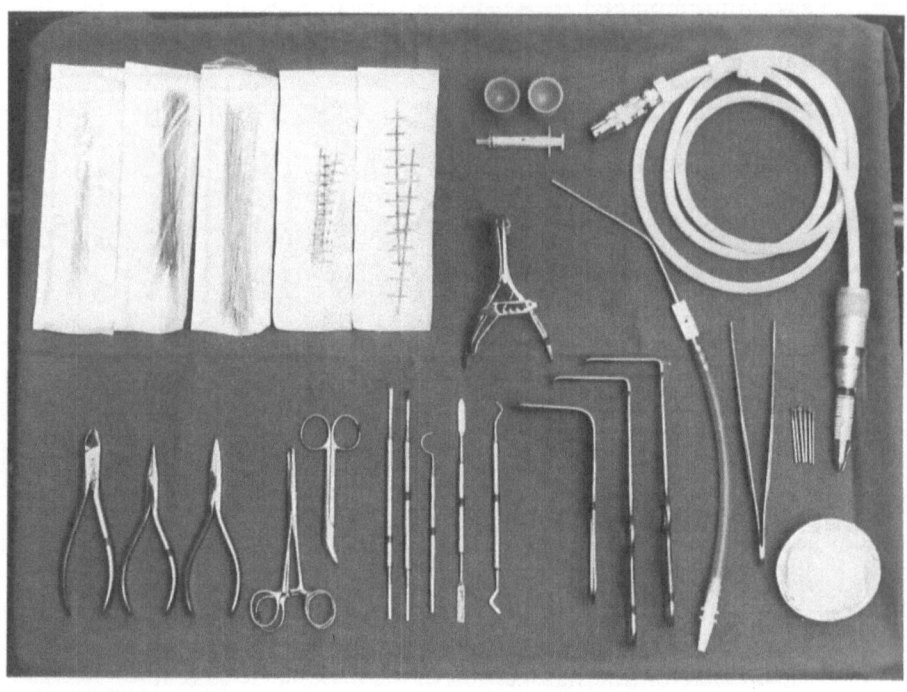

Fig. 23

Bottom (left to right):
1 Side-cutting forceps
1 Pointed forceps
1 Flat forceps
2 Bulldog forceps
1 Wire-cutting scissors, angled
1 Gauze packer, narrow
1 Gauze packer, broad
1 Dental probe
1 Cement spatula
1 Amalgam spatula
1 Tongue depressor
2 Langenbeck retractors
1 Fine suction tube with connecting
  tube
1 Tissue forceps
1 Basin with Vaseline strips
Connecting cable with micromotor,
handpiece, rose-head burrs and small
grindstone

Top (left to right):
Wires, 0.35 mm, 0.4 mm, 0.5 mm
4 Pediatric splints
2 Adult splints
1 Mouth gag
2 Rubber cups for acrylate
1 Syringe, 2 cm³

3.8.2 Instruments for Internal Fixation of the Maxilla

Indications:

- Central and lateral midfacial fractures, especially when comminuted or associated with bone loss.

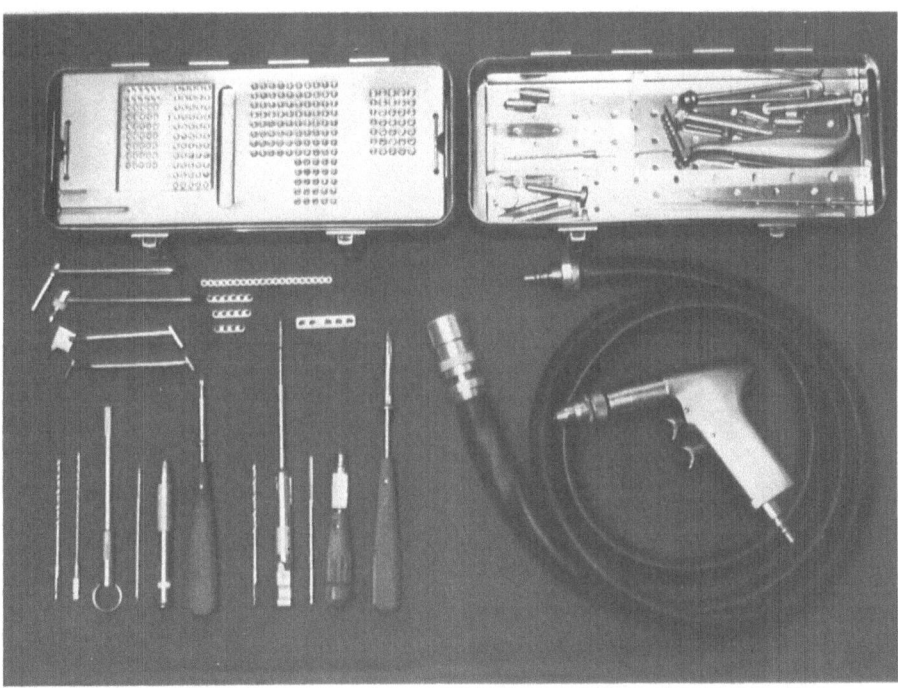

Fig. 24

Bottom (left to right):
Shown from the Basic Instrument Set
for Maxillofacial Bone Surgery:
1 Drill Bit, 2.0 mm
1 Drill Bit, 1.5 mm
1 Mini Depth Gauge, extra-long
1 Tap, 2.0 mm
1 Handle with mini quick coupling
1 Cruciform Screwdriver
1 Drill Bit, 2.7 mm
1 Small Depth Gauge, extra-long
1 Tap Sleeve, 2.7 mm
1 Handle with quick coupling
1 Small Screwdriver

Middle (left to right):
1 Tap Sleeve, 3.5 mm
1 Special DCP Drill Guide for Mandibular Plates
1 Drill Guide and Drill Sleeve
1 Mini Drill Sleeve, 1.1 and 1.5 mm

Shown from the implant set:
Straight Narrow Reconstruction Plate
Mini Plates (2.0 mm)
DCP, 2.7 mm
Small Air Drill
Air Hose

Top (left to right):
Implant and Basic Instrument Sets for
Maxillofacial Bone Surgery

3.8.3 Instruments for Internal Fixation of the Orbit

Indications:

- Fractures of the orbit.

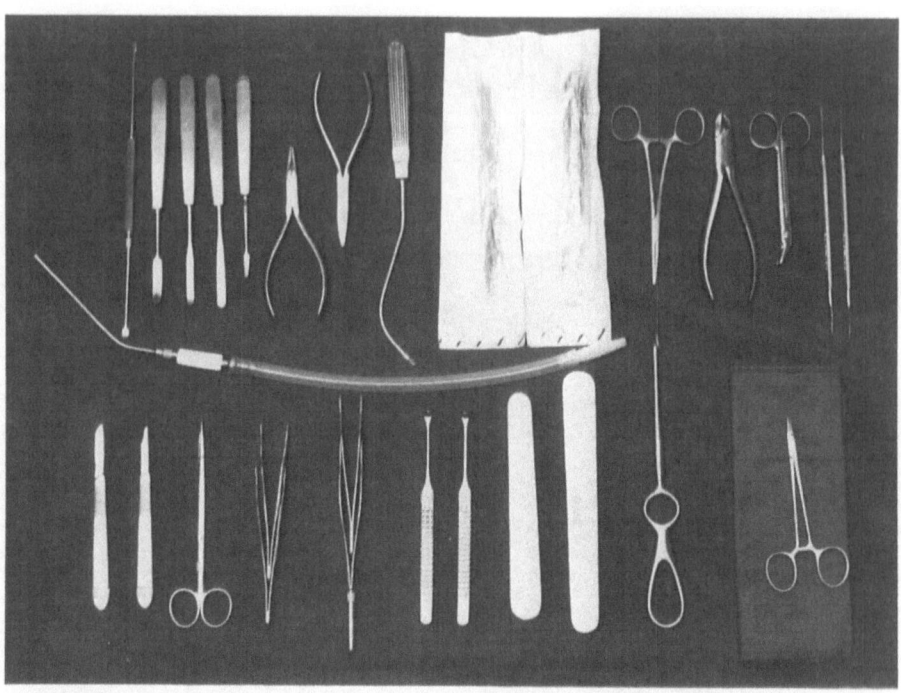

Fig. 25

Bottom (left to right):
2 Scalpels, nos. 10 and 15
1 Fine dissecting scissors
2 Fine surgical forceps
1 Coagulation forceps
1 Fine tissue forceps
2 Small Green retractors
2 Orbital spatulas
1 Simple hook
1 Needle holder, small

Middle:
1 Fine suction tube with connecting
  tube

Top (left to right):
1 Fine periosteal elevator, long
4 Periosteal elevators
1 Pointed forceps
1 Flat forceps
1 Curved awl
Wires, 0.35 mm, 0.4 mm, 0.5 mm
1 Bulldog forceps, straight
1 Side-cutting forceps
1 Wire-cutting scissors, angled
1 Gauze packer, narrow
1 Gauze packer, broad

3.8.4 Cranio Fixateur Externe

Indications:

- External fixation of midfacial fractures (see Figs. 27–30).

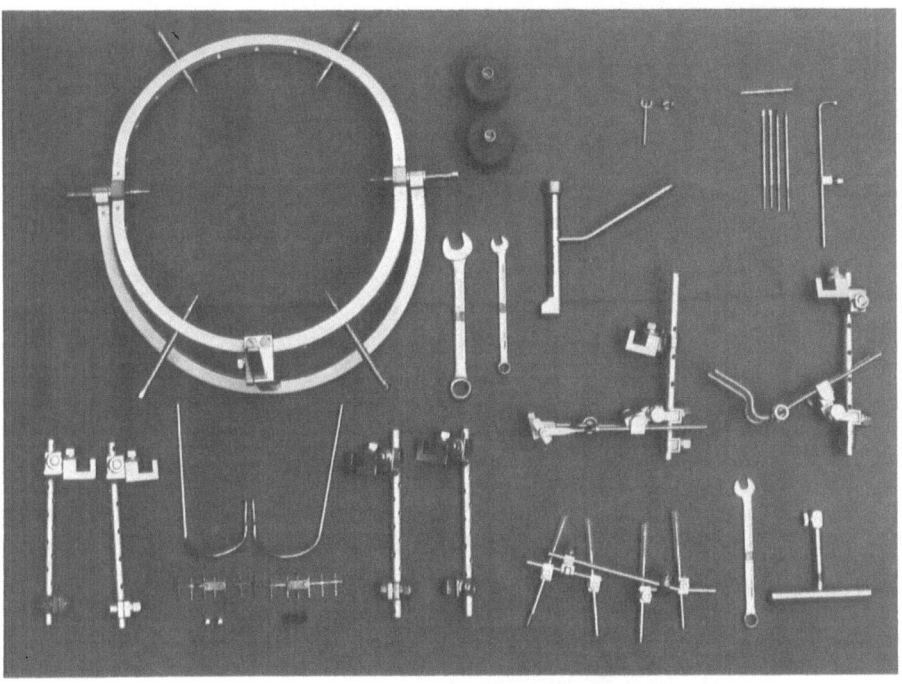

Fig. 26

Top (left):
1 Halo with Visor
Fixation Screws, 40 mm, 60 mm, 85 mm (2 each)
2 Socket Wrenches, 6 mm
1 Combination Wrench, 11 mm
1 Combination Wrench, 6 mm
1 Geared Socket Wrench, 90°, 6 mm across flats

Bottom (left):
4 Connecting Tubes, 7 mm
4 Suspending Clamps
4 Holding Clamps
Left and right Oral Rods, 1 each
1 Maxillary Arch Bar with 4 Nuts (only 2 shown)
2 Rubber Protection Caps

Top (right):
For zygomatic extension:
1 Extension Washer (for 2.7 mm screws)
3 Schanz Screws, 4 mm

Middle (right):
For nasal extension/fixation:
1) Extranasal fixation:
1 Suspending Clamp
1 Connecting Tube
1 Double Clamp with Hinge
1 Stop Clamp
1 Adjusting Screw
2 Nasal Plates

2) Intranasal fixation:
1 Suspending Clamp
1 Connecting Tube
1 Double Clamp with Hinge
1 Stop Clamp
1 Adjusting Screw
2 Nasal Rods

Bottom (right):
External Fixator
Combination Wrench, 7 mm
Handle for Schanz Screws and Steinmann Pins

3.9 Use of the Cranio Fixateur Externe for Various Midfacial Fractures

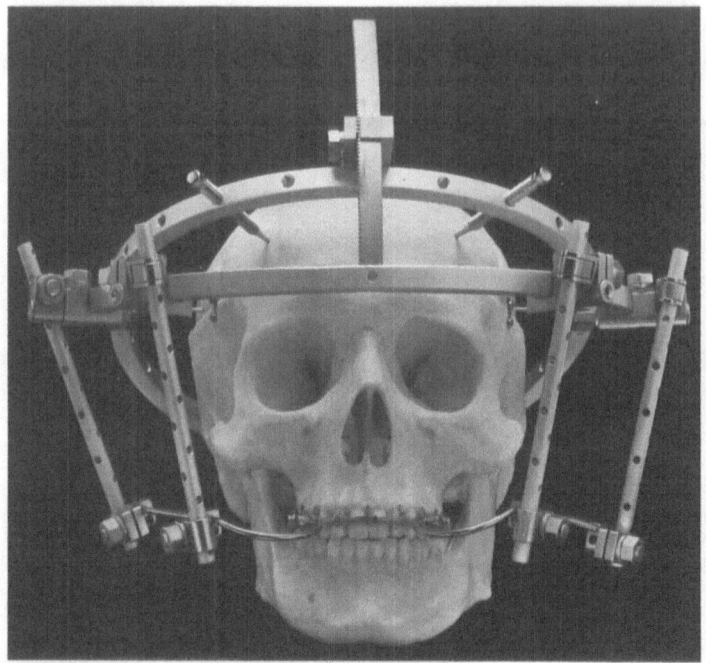

Fig. 27.
Fixation of a
mandibular
fracture with
the Cranio Fi-
xateur externe

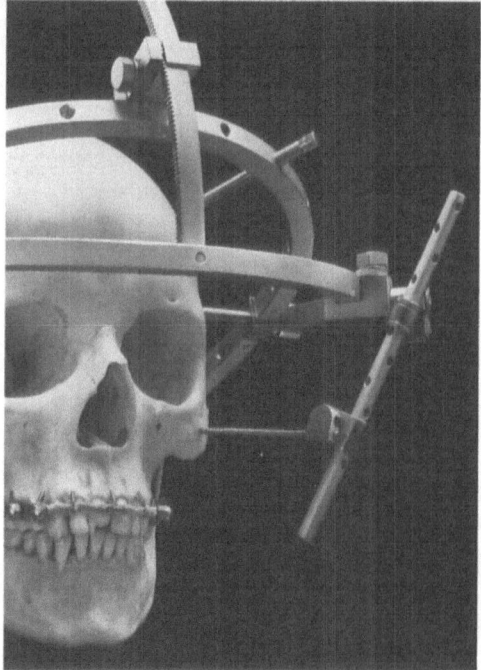

Fig. 28. Zygomatic extension with
a Schanz screw

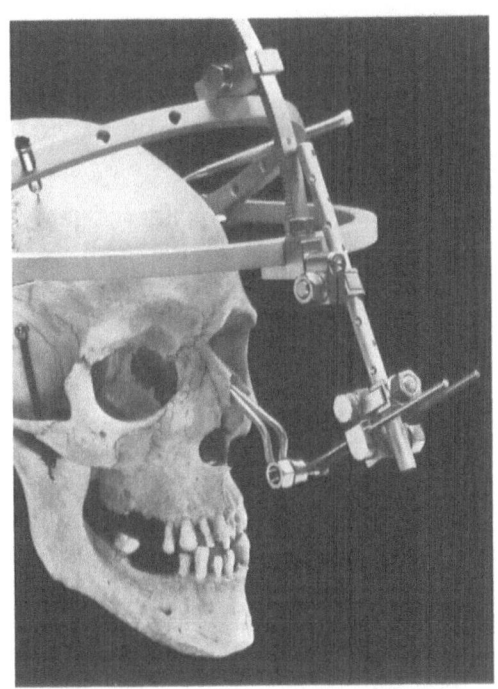

Fig. 29. Intranasal fixation

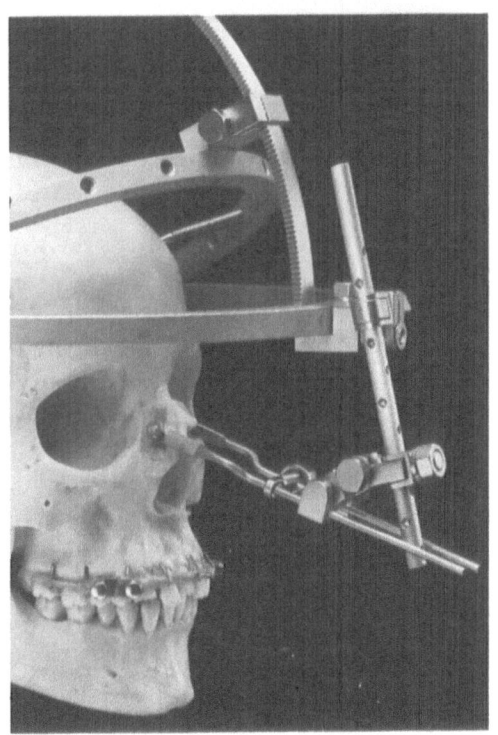

Fig. 30. Extranasal fixation

3.10 Operative Procedure

- The pharynx is packed with Vaseline strips; the lips are smeared with Vaseline.

- Arch bars and intermaxillary fixation are applied.

- Intubation line is brought across chin to left arm.

- Patient is redraped.

- The fracture is exposed at the lateral and caudal orbital rim.

- The fracture is reduced with bone hooks.

- Fixation is carried out with wire ligatures.

- Comminuted fractures and fractures with bone loss can often be fixed with mini zygomatic plates or adaption plates.
    - Afer reduction, holes are drilled near the fracture with the 1.5 mm drill bit and mini drill sleeve.
    - The necessary screw length is measured.
    - The thread is cut (2.0 mm tap).
    - Cortex screws, 2.0 mm, are inserted.

- Orbital floor defects are repaired with lyophilized dura or silicone sheeting.

- The wound is closed.
    - Muscle: absorbable 5/0
    - Mucosa: nonabsorbable 4/0, braided
    - Skin: nonabsorbable 5/0, continuous intracutaneous

- A spray dressing is applied to the wound, followed by adhesive strips.

- The cranio Fixateur externe is applied:
    - The halo with visor is held in place by two posterior screws inserted above the attachment of the neck muscles, two frontal screws inserted above the frontal hairline, and two lateral screws, which are the last to be inserted. The visor part of the halo is parallel to the bipupillary line, and the whole system is centered on the midline.
    - Using the geared socket wrench, each of the two oral rods is attached to the maxillary arch bar with two screws.
    The oral rods are bent so that they fit comfortably in the corners of the mouth.
    - The oral rods are connected to the visor by means of two external fixation elements consisting of suspending clamps, connecting tubes and holding clamps (see Fig. 27).

- If a nasal fracture is also present (see Figs. 29 and 30, p. 35)
    - Nasal bones are reduced and fixed with plaster and packing.

- Saddle nose is corrected by intranasal fixation device connected to visor.
- Broad nose is corrected by extranasal fixation device connected to visor.

- An unstable, comminuted zygomatic fracture may require additional fixation of the zygoma (see Figs. 28, p. 34):
  - Fixation with Schanz screws attached to outrigger on visor.

3.11 Postoperative Care

- Reduction of swelling: – Cold, moist compresses.

- Oral hygiene:
  - After meals spray oral cavity thoroughly with antiseptic solution.
  - Start normal tooth brushing, followed by antiseptic rinse, as soon as possible.
  - Smear lips with Vaseline.
  - Air humidifier.

- Mobilization:
  - According to surgeon's orders; will depend on patient's general condition (cerebral, pulmonary).

- Antibiotics: – As ordered.

- Check roentgenograms: – Before discharge.

- Hospitalization time:
  - About 1 week for midfacial fractures;
  - Longer for multiple injuries.

- Suture removal:
  - If healing is progressing well:
    - facial sutures are removed on 4th or 5th day;
    - neck sutures after 7–10 days;
    - intraoral mucosal sutures are removed after 2–3 weeks.

- Cranio Fixateur externe: – Remains in place for 6–8 weeks.

- Follow-up examinations: – Weekly or biweekly.

- Removal of wire ligatures: – After 6 months, under local anesthesia.

4 Orthognathic Maxillofacial Surgery

4.1 Indications

Dysgnathias: Deformities of the jaws, including:
a) Prognathism and retrognathism of the maxilla.
b) Prognathism and retrognathism of the mandible (progenia and microgenia).
c) Open bite or overbite deformity.
d) Protrusion or retrusion of teeth.

4.2 Principle and Goals

- An osteotomy is done through one segment of the dental arch (*segmental osteotomy*), through the entire mandible (corpus or ramus osteotomies, i.e. *sagittal split osteotomy*), or through the entire maxilla (*Le Fort osteotomy*).

- The osteotomized fragment is moved to the desired position.

- Functionally stable fixation is carried out (splinting, lag screw fixation, plating, cranial external fixation).

4.3 Workup Materials that are Taken into Surgery

- Plaster models: Original models, simulation models.

- Simulographic study.

- Photographs of the face and dental arch.

- Roentgenograms: Teleroentgenograms, orthopantogram, and possibly dental films.

4.4 Preparation of the Patient on the Day Before Surgery

- Dental calculus is removed.
- Dental splints are applied.
- Individual teeth are ground as needed.
- Mouth is rinsed with antiseptic solution every 2 hours.

4.5 Preoperative Preparation of the Patient

- Anesthesia:
  - Nasal intubation with line passed over forehead to left arm.
  - Nasogastric tube.
  - Urinary catheter and heated mattress (if anesthesia is prolonged).

- Positioning:
  - Head freely movable and accessible from both sides and from above (surgeon + two assistants).
  - Inflatable cushion under shoulders.

- Preparation of operative site:
  - Spray oral cavity with antiseptic solution.
  - Do skin disinfection of face and neck.
  - Drape the patient as for thyroid surgery, with the mouth draped free.

4.6 Instruments and Equipment to be Prepared

- Splint and template, stored in antiseptic solution.
- Instrument trays for facial bone surgery.
- Splinting instrument set (for segmental osteotomy).
- AO/ASIF basic instrument set and implant set for maxillofacial bone surgery (for sagittal splitting).
- Cranio Fixateur externe (for Le Fort osteotomy).
- Dental drill.

- Pressurized sprayer.

- Head light for surgeon.

- Suture material
  - Mucosa: nonabsorbable 4/0, braided
  - Skin: nonabsorbable 5/0

4.7 Table Setups for Orthognathic Maxillofacial Surgery

- Instruments for splinting (see 4.7.1)

- Setup (1st table) for exposing the osteotomy site (see 4.7.2)

- Setup (2nd table) for performing the osteotomy and carrying out trans-buccal fixation (see 4.7.3)

- Instruments for internal fixation of the orbit (see 4.7.4)

- Instruments for internal fixation of the maxilla (see 4.7.5)

- Cranio Fixateur externe (see 4.7.6)

4.7.1 Instruments for Splinting

Indications:

- Segmental osteotomy.

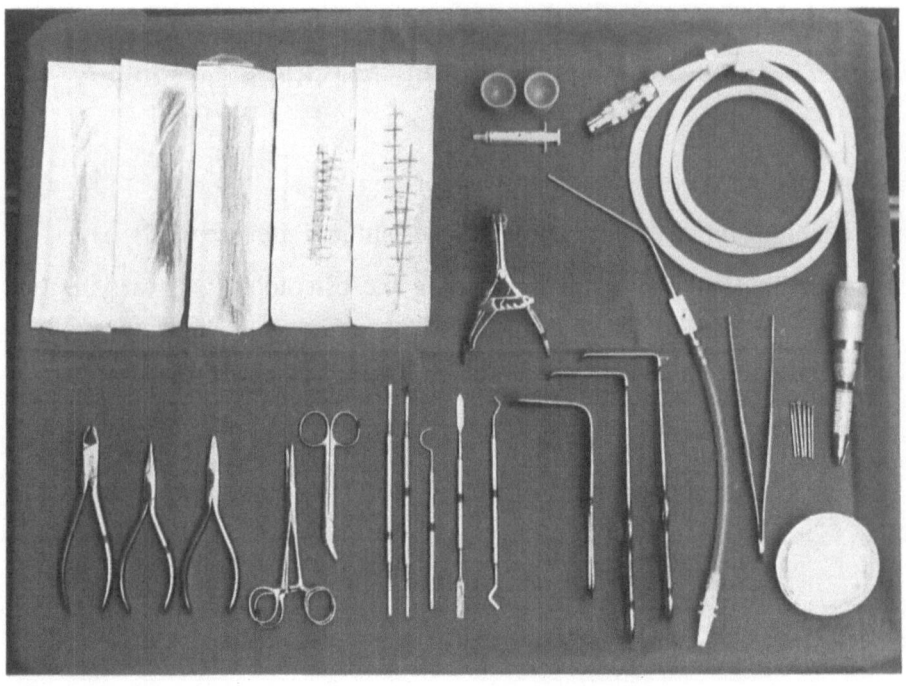

Fig. 31

Bottom (left to right):
1 Side-cutting forceps
1 Pointed forceps
1 Flat forceps
2 Bulldog forceps
1 Wire-cutting scissors, angled
1 Gauze packer, narrow
1 Gauze packer, broad
1 Dental probe
1 Cement spatula
1 Amalgam spatula
1 Tongue depressor
2 Langenbeck retractors
1 Fine suction tube with connecting tube
1 Tissue forceps
1 Basin with Vaseline strips
Connecting cable with micromotor, handpiece, rose-head burrs and small grindstone

Top (left to right):
Wires, 0.35 mm, 0.4 mm, 0.5 mm
4 Pediatric splints
2 Adult splints
1 Mouth gag
2 Rubber cups for acrylate
1 Syringe, 2 cm³

4.7.2 Instruments for Orthognathic Maxillofacial Surgery (1st Table)

Indications:

- Exposure of osteotomy site for corpus or ramus osteotomy, Le Fort osteotomy, segmental osteotomy.

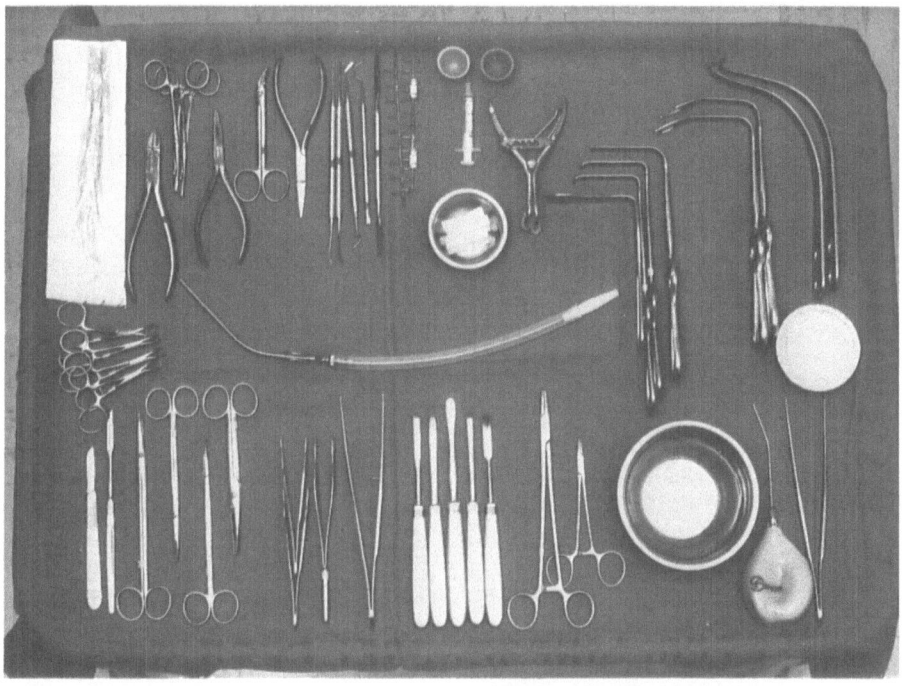

Fig. 32

Bottom (left to right):
2 Scalpels, nos. 10 and 15
3 Fine dissecting scissors
1 Mayo scissors
1 Fine surgical forceps (extraoral)
1 Fine tissue forceps (extraoral)
1 Fine surgical forceps (intraoral)
5 Periosteal elevators
1 Needle holder, long (intraoral)
1 Needle holder, short (extraoral)
1 Basin for irrigating solution
1 Irrigating bulb
1 Tissue forceps
1 Basin for Vaseline strips

Middle (left to right):
4 Towel clamps
1 Suction tube with connecting tube

Top (left to right):
Wires, 0.35 mm, 0.4 mm, 0.5 mm
1 Side-cutting forceps

2 Bulldog forceps
1 Pointed forceps
1 Wire-cutting scissors, angled
1 Flat forceps
1 Gauze packer, narrow
1 Gauze packer, broad
1 Amalgam spatula
1 Dental probe
1 Cement spatula
2 Splints for maxilla and mandible
2 Rubber cups for acrylate
1 Syringe, 2 cm³
1 Basin with cotton rolls
1 Tongue depressor
2 Langenbeck retractors
   (or: 2 Langenbeck retractors, short
   and 2 Langenbeck retractors, long)
1 Swallowtail Retractor
2 Forked Retractors, left and right
1 Internal Retractor, narrow
1 External Retractor, broad

43

4.7.3 Instruments for Orthognathic Maxillofacial Surgery (2nd Table)

Indications:

- All osteotomies for bone division.

- Osteotomy of the ramus (sagittal split) and body of the mandible for trans-buccal internal fixation.

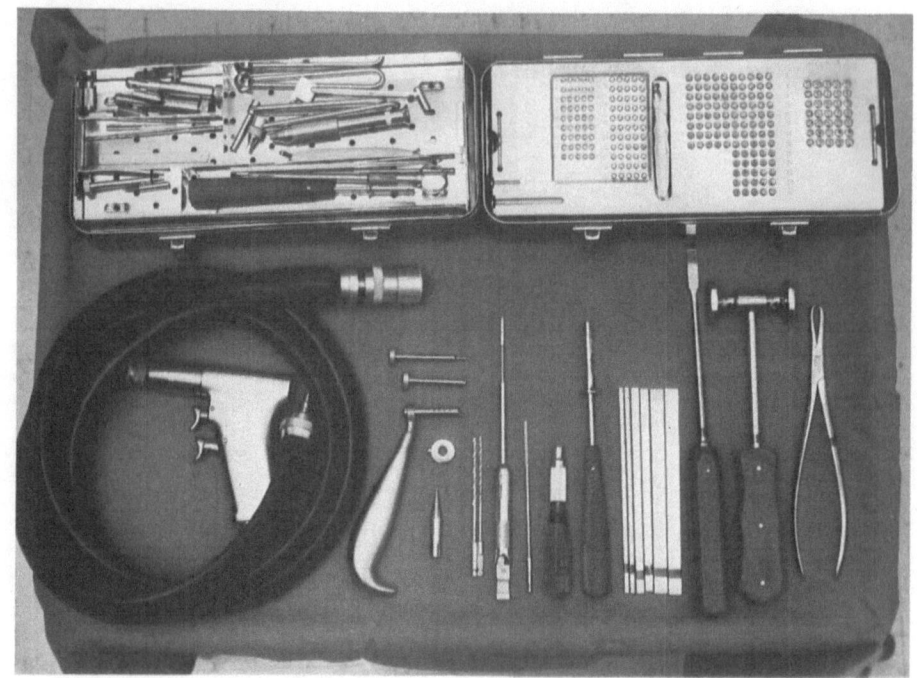

Fig. 33

Bottom (left to right):
1 Small Air Drill
1 Air Hose
Shown from Basic Instrument Set for
Maxillofacial Bone Surgery:
1 Trocar with handle
1 Mountable Ring/Cheek Retractor
1 Trocar point, large
1 Drill Sleeve, 2.0 mm
1 Drill Sleeve, 2.7 mm
1 Drill Bit, 2.7 mm
1 Drill Bit, 2.0 mm
1 Small Depth Gauge, extra-long

1 Tap, 2.7 mm
1 Handle with quick coupling
1 Small Screwdriver
Osteotomes, 2 mm, 5 mm, 10 mm
(2 each)
1 Long chisel
1 Hammer
1 Bone holding forceps

Top (left to right):
Basic Instrument Set for Maxillofacial
Bone Surgery
Implant Set for Mandibular Surgery

4.7.4 Instruments for Internal Fixation of the Orbit

Indications:

- Osteotomies of the orbit.

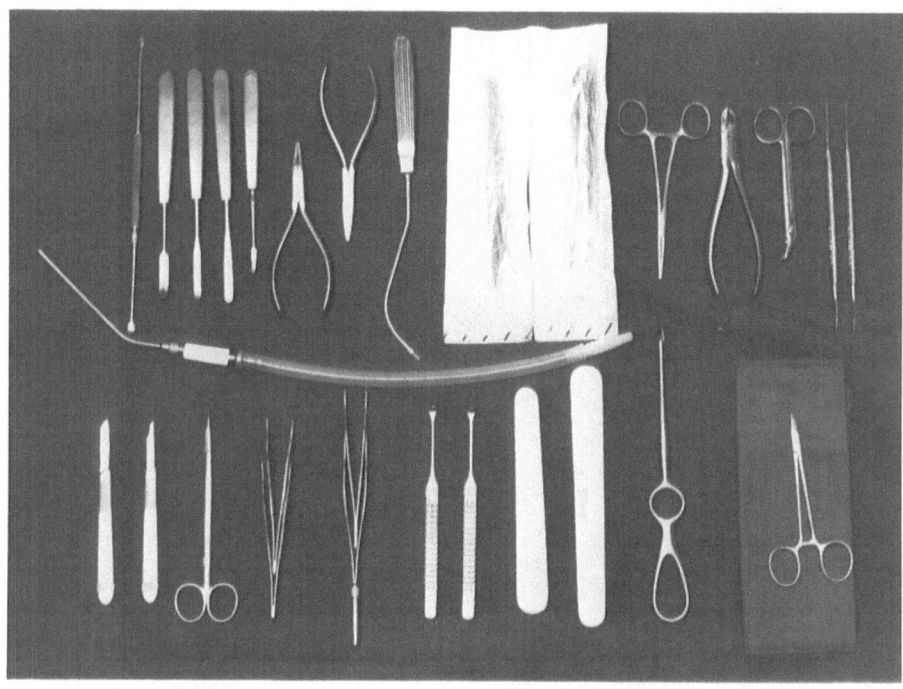

Fig. 34

Bottom (left to right):
2 Scalpels, nos. 10 and 15
1 Fine dissecting scissors
2 Fine surgical forceps
1 Coagulation forceps
1 Fine tissue forceps
2 Small Green retractors
2 Orbital spatulas
1 Simple hook
1 Needle holder, small

Middle:
1 Fine suction tube with connecting
  tube

Top (left to right):
1 Fine periosteal elevator, long
4 Periosteal elevators
1 Pointed forceps
1 Flat forceps
1 Curved awl
Wires, 0.35 mm, 0.4 mm, 0.5 mm
1 Forceps, straight
1 Side-cutting forceps
1 Wire-cutting scissors, angled
1 Gauze packer, narrow
1 Gauze packer, broad

4.7.5 Instruments for Internal Fixation of the Maxilla

Indications:

- Le Fort osteotomies, and possibly segmental osteotomies.

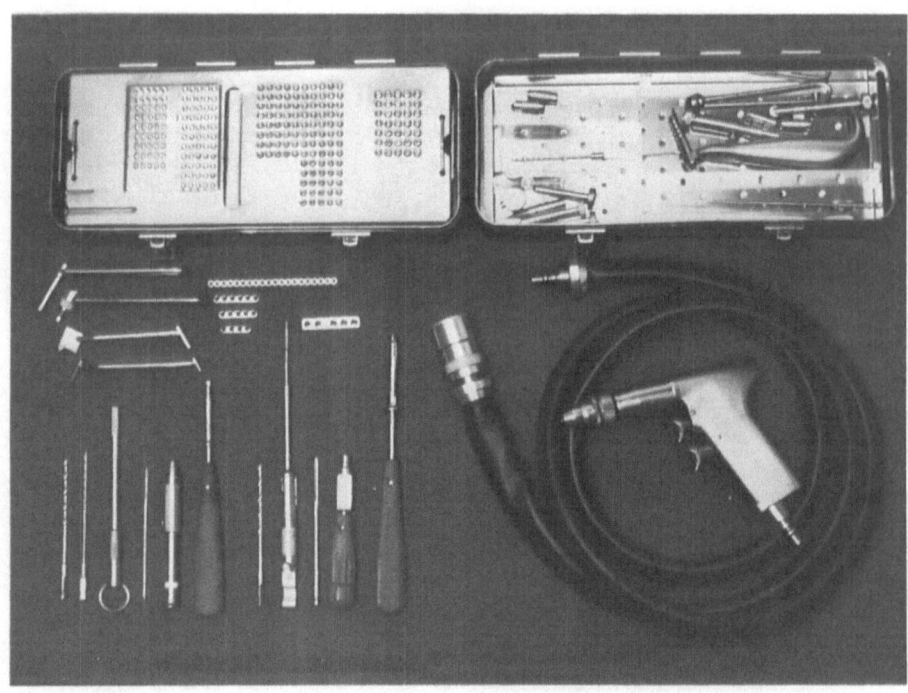

Fig. 35

Bottom (left to right):
Shown from the Basic Instrument Set
for Maxillofacial Bone Surgery:
1 Drill Bit, 2.0 mm
1 Drill Bit, 1.5 mm
1 Mini Depth Gauge, extra-long
1 Tap, 2.0 mm
1 Handle with mini quick coupling
1 Cruciform Screwdriver
1 Drill Bit, 2.7 mm
1 Small Depth Gauge, extra-long
1 Tap, 2.7 mm
1 Handle with quick coupling
1 Small Screwdriver

Middle (left to right):
1 Tap Sleeve, 3.5 mm
1 Special DCP Drill Guide for Mandibular Plates
1 Drill Sleeve and Drill Guide
1 Mini Drill Sleeve, 1.1 mm and 1.5 mm

Shown from the implant set:
Straight Narrow Reconstruction Plate
Mini Plates, 2.0 mm
DCP, 2.7 mm
Small Air Drill
Air Hose

Top (left to right):
Implant and Basic Instrument Sets for
Maxillofacial Bone Surgery

4.7.6 Cranio Fixateur Externe

Indications:

- Le Fort osteotomy, osteotomy of the zygoma and nasal skeleton (e.g., for saddle nose; see Fig. 37).

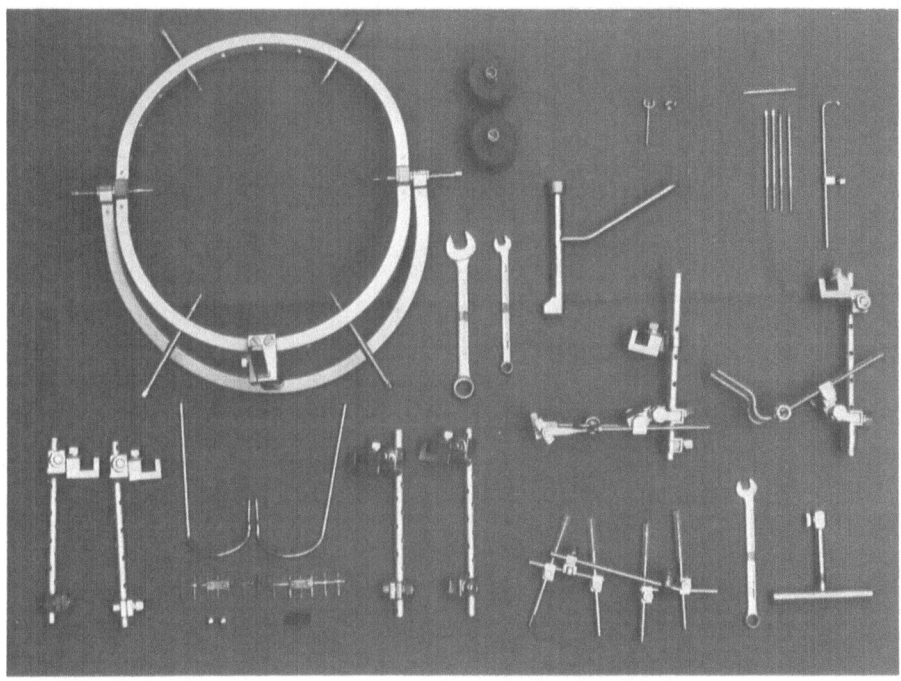

Fig. 36

Top (left):
1 Halo with Visor
Fixation Screws, 40 mm, 60 mm, 85 mm
(2 each)
2 Socket Wrenches
1 Combination Wrench, 11 mm
1 Combination Wrench, 6 mm
1 Geared Socket Wrench, 90°, 6 mm
across flats

Bottom (left):
4 Connecting Tubes, 7 mm
4 Suspending Clamps
4 Holding Clamps
2 Oral Rods, left and right
1 Maxillary Arch Bar with 4 Nuts
2 Protection Caps, rubber (only 1
shown)

Top (right):
For zygomatic extension:
1 Extension washer (for 2.7 mm screws)
4 Schanz Screws, 4 mm
1 Stop Clamp

Middle (right):
For nasal extension/fixation

1) Extranasal fixation:
1 Suspending Clamp
1 Connecting Tube
1 Double Clamp with Hinge
1 Stop Clamp
1 Adjusting Screw
2 Nasal Plates

2) Intranasal fixation:
1 Suspending Clamp
1 Connecting Tube
1 Double Clamp with Hinge
1 Stop Clamp
1 Adjusting Screw
2 Nasal Rods

Bottom (right):
External Fixator
Combination Wrench, 7 mm
Handle for Schanz Screws and Steinmann Pins

47

4.8 Examples of Various Osteotomies

4.8.1 Correction Within the Dental Arch

Mandible   **Maxilla**

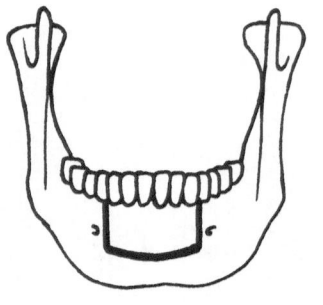

a Segmental osteotomy of the mandible

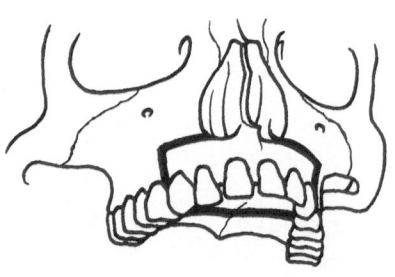

d Frontal segmental osteotomy of the maxilla

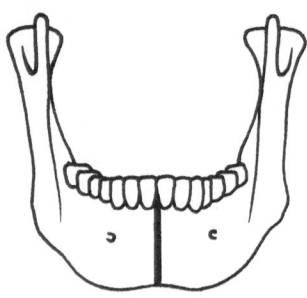

b Symphyseal osteotomy

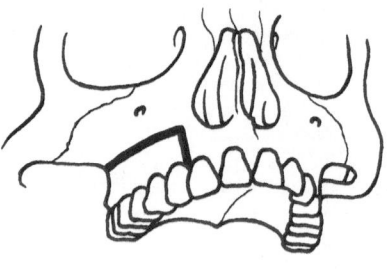

e Unilateral segmental osteotomy

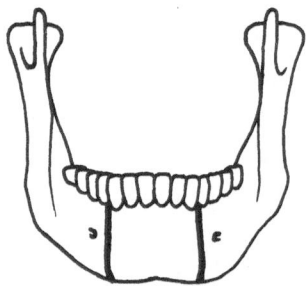

c Bilateral corpus osteotomy

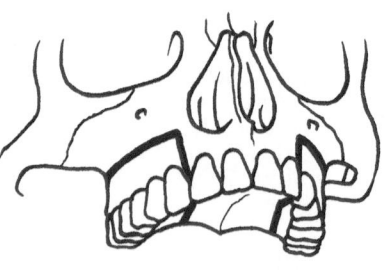

f Bilateral segmental osteotomy

Fig. 37 a–h. Osteotomies of the maxilla and mandible

4.8.2 Correction Outside the Dental Arch

Mandible

Maxilla

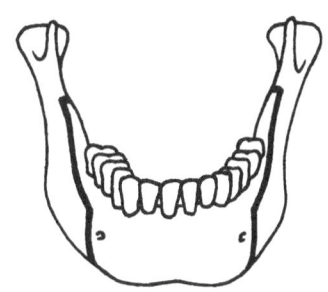

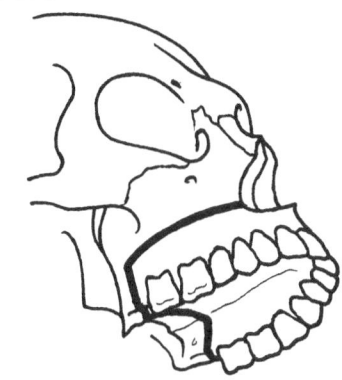

Fig. 37 g. Sagittal split osteotomy

Fig. 37 h. Le Fort I osteotomy

4.9 Operative Procedure

- Pharynx is packed with Vaseline strips.
- Lips are smeared with Vaseline.
- A vasoconstrictor is infiltrated locally to control hemorrhage.

4.9.1 Further Procedure for a Segmental Osteotomy

- The segmental osteotomy is performed from the vestibular and palatine sides with a dental drill.
- The segments are mobilized.
- The mucosa is sutured with size 4/0, nonabsorbable.
- For fixation, the acrylic template and splint prepared from the simulation model are wired into place. The acrylate template is stored in antiseptic solution at the start of the operation and is used to secure accurate positioning as well as to augment the fixation.

4.9.2 Further Procedure for Sagittal Splitting

- The patient is placed in the reverse Trendelenburg position.
- The ascending ramus of the mandible is exposed through an intraoral approach.
- Sagittal splitting is done with a dental drill (see Fig. 37).
- The same is done on the opposite side.
- The mandible is mobilized into the desired occlusal position.
- The jaws are fixed with intermaxillary wires.
- The fragments are fixed with three lag screws per side, inserted transbuccally (see Fig. 38).
- The intermaxillary wires are removed.
- Redon drains are inserted on each side.
- The oral cavity is sprayed thoroughly with antiseptic solution.
- The wound is closed:
  - Mucosa: nonabsorbable 4/0, braided
  - Skin: nonabsorbable 5/0
- A spray dressing is applied to the wound, followed by adhesive bandage strips.

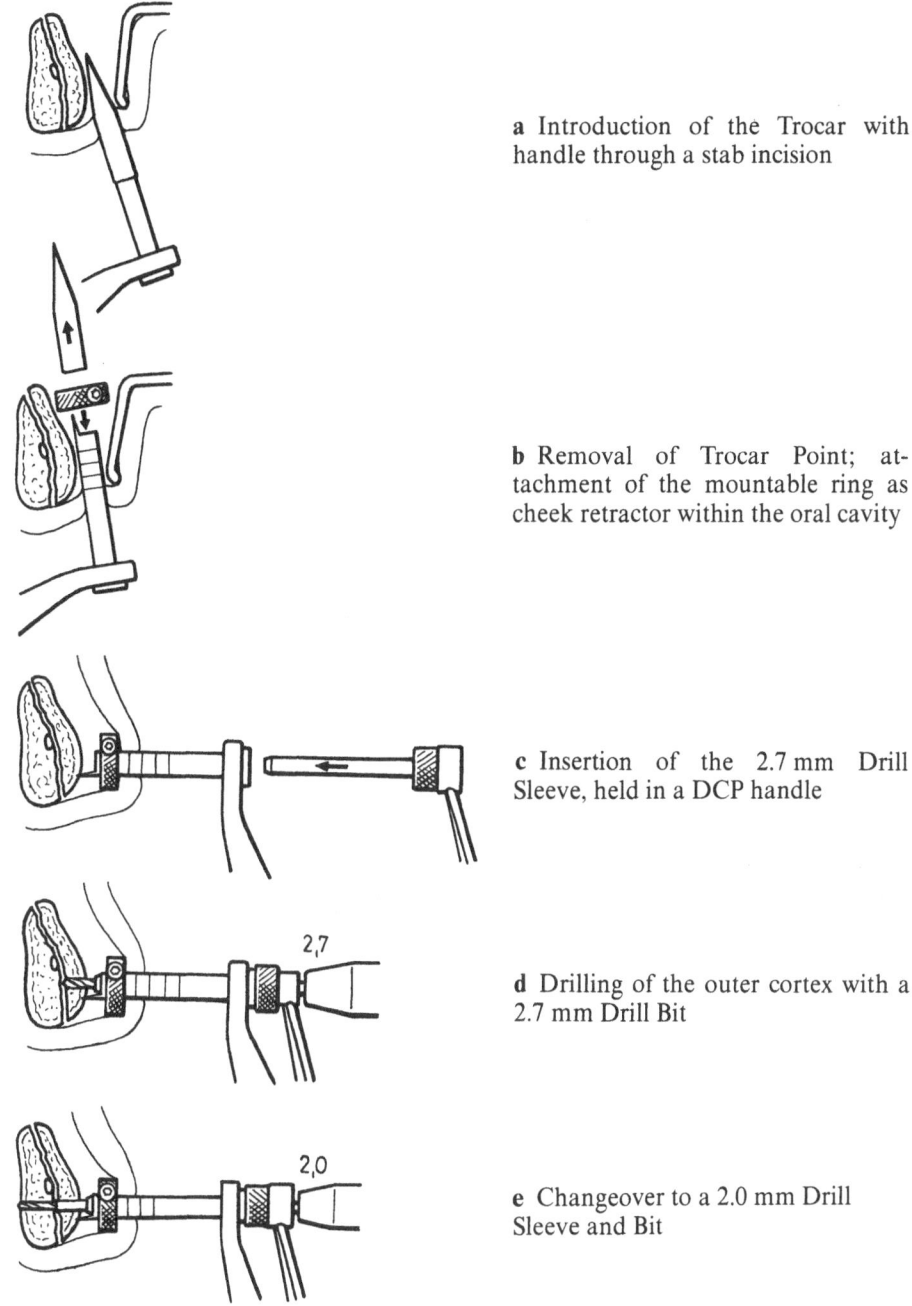

a Introduction of the Trocar with handle through a stab incision

b Removal of Trocar Point; attachment of the mountable ring as cheek retractor within the oral cavity

c Insertion of the 2.7 mm Drill Sleeve, held in a DCP handle

d Drilling of the outer cortex with a 2.7 mm Drill Bit

e Changeover to a 2.0 mm Drill Sleeve and Bit

Fig. 38 a–i. Transbuccal fixation of mandibular fragments by means of three lag screws per side

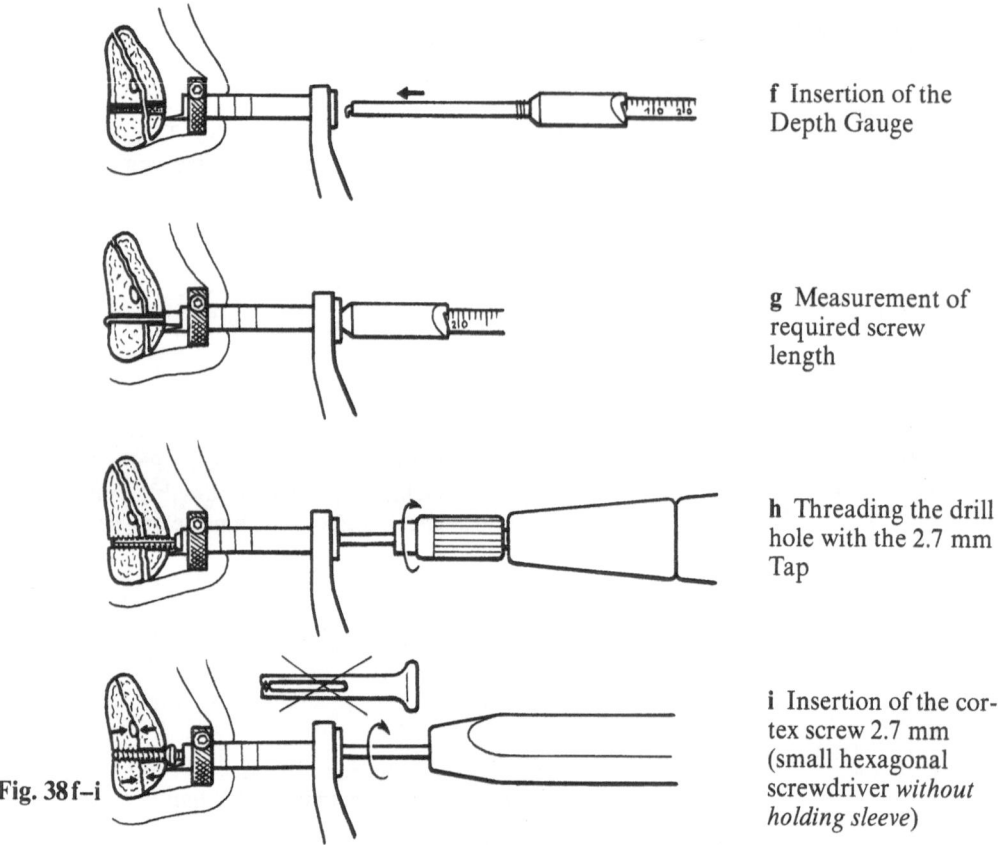

f Insertion of the Depth Gauge

g Measurement of required screw length

h Threading the drill hole with the 2.7 mm Tap

Fig. 38 f–i

i Insertion of the cortex screw 2.7 mm (small hexagonal screwdriver *without holding sleeve*)

4.9.3 Further Procedure for a Le Fort I Osteotomy

- A vertical mucosal incision is made in the vestibule.

- The gingival mucosa is incised.

- A vestibular and palatal osteotomy is performed with a dental drill.

- The maxilla is mobilized into the desired occlusal position.

- The mucosa is sutured with nonabsorbable 4/0, braided.

- For a Le Fort I osteotomy involving several segments of the maxilla, the prepared acrylic template and maxillary arch bar are wired into place at this time. (For a standard Le Fort I osteotomy, splints are applied preoperatively.)

- The jaws are fixed with intermaxillary wires.

- Cranio fixateur externe is applied:
  - The halo with visor is held in place by two posterior screws inserted above the attachment of the neck muscles, two frontal screws inserted above the frontal hairline, and two lateral screws, which are the last to be inserted. The visor part of the halo is parallel to the bipupillary line, and the whole system is centered on the midline.
  - The two oral rods are apposed to the maxillary arch bar and bent so that they fit comfortably in the corners of the mouth. Using the 90° geared socket wrench, the oral rods are attached to the arch bar with 2 screws per side and tightened with the 6 mm combination wrench.
  - The external fixation elements are applied: The oral rods are connected to the visor by means of 2 suspending clamps, 2 connecting tubes and 2 holding clamps per side (see Fig. 27, p. 34).

- The intermaxillary wires are removed.

After a segmental or Le Fort I osteotomy:

- Remove pharyngeal pack.

- Smear lips with Vaseline.

4.10 Postoperative Care

- Reduction of swelling: – Cold, moist compresses

- Oral hygiene:
  - After meals spray oral cavity thoroughly with antiseptic solution.
  - Start normal tooth brushing, followed by antiseptic rinse, as soon as possible.
  - Smear lips with Vaseline.
  - Air humidifier.

- Mobilization: – As ordered.

- Antibiotics: – As ordered.

- Check roentgenograms: – Before discharge.

- Hospitalization time: – About 1 week.

- Suture removal:
  - If healing is progressing well:
  - facial sutures are removed on 4th or 5th day;
  - neck sutures after 7–10 days;
  - intraoral mucosal sutures are removed after 2–3 weeks.

- Cranio Fixateur externe: – Remains in place for 6–8 weeks.

- Follow-up examinations: – Every 1–2 weeks.

- Removal of screws: – After about 18 months.

5 AO/ASIF Instruments for Maxillofacial Bone Surgery

102.62*

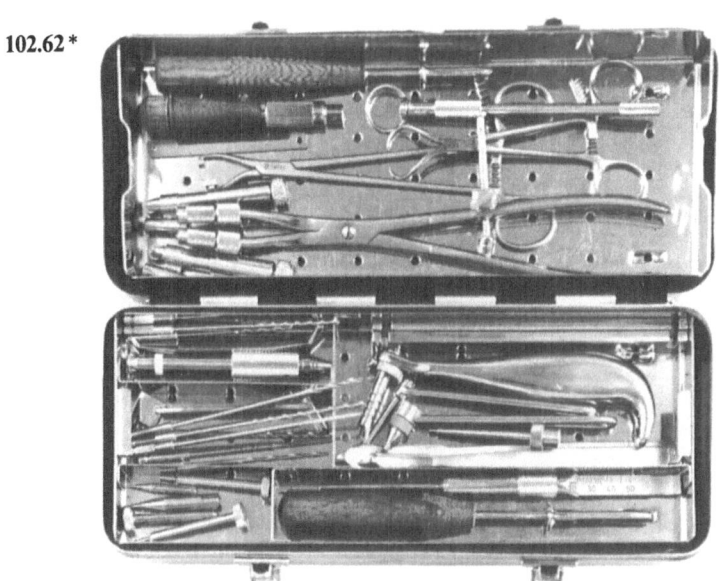

* "SYNTHES" Catalogue number

5.1 Instruments for 2.7 mm dia. Screws

310.19

Drill Bit, 2.0 mm

with end to fit quick coupling of small air drill. Used to drill the threaded hole for 2.7 mm cortex screws and the gliding hole for 2.0 mm cortex screws.

310.21

Long drill bit for transbuccal drilling through the trocar with handle.

310.26

Drill Bit, 2.7 mm

with end to fit quick coupling of small air drill. Used to drill the gliding hole for 2.7 mm cortex screws.

310.28

Long drill bit for transbuccal drilling through the trocar with handle.

311.26

Tap, 2.7 mm

with end to fit quick coupling of tap handle. Used to cut the thread for 2.7 mm cortex screws.

311.28

Extra-long tap for transbuccal drilling through the trocar with handle.

310.81

Long countersink

with interchangeable centering sleeve for 2.7 mm and 2.0 mm screws. Used to cut a recess for the screw head.
Can be used with the transbuccal trocar.

311.43

Handle with quick coupling

receives the 2.7 mm tap. The movable end-piece of the handle can be braced against the palm for better working precision.

312.20

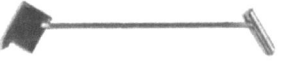

Drill Guide and Drill Sleeve 2.0 mm

for use with the 2.0 mm drill bit. The spiked end is used on bare bone; the round end is for use on ¼-tubular plates. The drill sleeve can be slid over a preplaced Kirschner wire, enabling a hole to be drilled parallel to the wire.

312.26

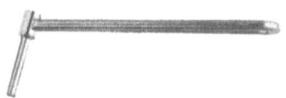

Tap Sleeve, 3.5 mm

protects tissues when the 2.7 mm tap is used.

322.24

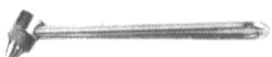

Special DCP Drill Guide for Mandibular Plates

receives the 2.0 mm drill bit. For high-eccentricity drilling, the drill guide is placed on the side of the plate hole away from the fracture, with the 0.8 arrow pointing toward the fracture. For low-eccentricity drilling, the guide is positioned near the fracture with the 0.8 arrow pointing toward the fracture line.

This feature is important for screw placement in the transverse holes of the EDCP: high eccentricity is needed for the wide, dentulous jaw, while low eccentricity is best for the narrow, edentulous, atrophic jaw.

The hole can be centered by positioning the drill guide away from the fracture, with the 0 arrow pointing toward the fracture line.

The diameter of the drill guide is slightly less than that of the plate hole, enabling it to be used even at sites where the plate is strongly contoured.

322.25

Special DCP Drill Guide, long

used for DCP holes, like 322.24. Advantageous for deep drilling, like that required in tension-band plating of the mandibular angle.

322.24

The guide is used as described above, with or without a **handle,** and can be used with the transbuccal trocar.

319.08

Small Depth Gauge, extra-long

used to measure the necessary length of 2.7 mm (or possibly 3.5 mm) cortex screws. Also compatible with the transbuccal trocar.

314.02

Small Hexagonal Screwdriver, width across flats 2.5 mm

for insertion and removal of 2.7 mm (and 3.5 mm) cortex screws. When used through the trocar with handle, the holding sleeve for screws must be removed.

397.20

Small **Trocar Point** for screwdriver enables transbuccal screws to be removed from lateral part of jaw through a stab incision.

329.55
329.57

Bending Templates

made of aluminum, are easily molded to bone contours to provide a model for the contouring of plates.

329.04
329.05

Bending Irons

used to twist mandibular plates. They should not be used for bending (cf. Bending Pliers).

58

397.11

Trocar with handle and accessories

used for internal fixations of the lateral jaw during intraoral surgery (internal fixation of simple fractures, ramus and corpus osteotomies, screw fixation of DCP implants).

The trocar is introduced through a small stab incision, using the large **Metal point.** Once inside the mouth, the point is removed with a towel clamp, and the **Mountable Ring** as cheeck retractor is mounted on the trocar using the small screwdriver.

397.12

397.13

397.15

The trocar has a rotating sleeve with a sharp spike that engages securely against the bone.

Drilling is done through one of the three **Drill Sleeves** (1.5, 2.0 or 2.7 mm) or the long DCP drill guide. After the drill guide is removed, the trocar provides a stable channel for screw length gauging, tapping, and screw insertion.

397.16

397.17

5.2 Instruments for 2.0 mm dia. Screws

310.15   **Drill Bit, 1.5 mm**

with end to fit quick coupling of small air drill. Used to drill the threaded hole for the 2.0 mm screw and the gliding hole for a 1.5 mm lag screw.

310.16   Long drill bit designed for use through the trocar with handle.

311.19   **Tap with mini quick coupling, 2.0 mm**

Used to cut the thread for 2.0 mm cortex screws.

311.21   Long tap for use with the trocar with handle. Taps snap into the handle with mini quick coupling.

310.95   **Handle with mini quick coupling**

for use with 2.0 mm tap.

312.15   **Mini Drill Sleeve, 1.1 and 1.5 mm**

for use with 1.1 mm and 1.5 mm drill bits. Can be used on bare bone or in plate holes.

319.07   **Mini Depth Gauge, extra-long**

for measuring required length of 2.0 mm cortex screws; can be used through trocar with handle.

313.99

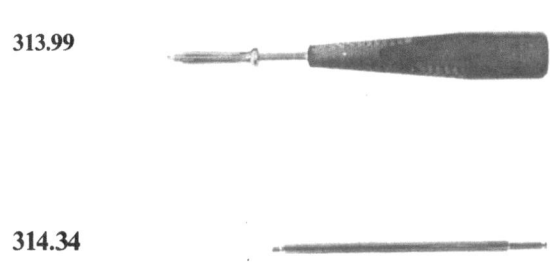

Cruciform Screwdriver

necessary for insertion of 2.0 mm cortex screws with cruciform slot. Can be used through trocar with handle after holding sleeve is removed.

314.34

The **Mini Hexagonal Screwdriver** 1.5 mm is used with the handle with mini quick coupling for insertion of the new 2.0 mm cortex screws with hexagonal socket.
Can be used through trocar with handle.

5.3 General Instruments

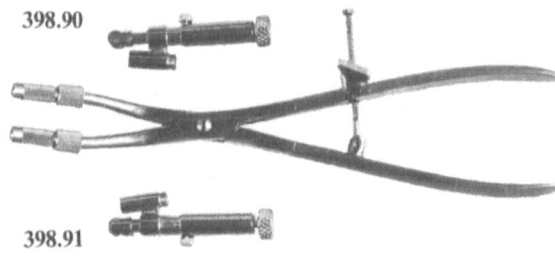

398.90

398.91

Mandibular Reduction Forceps

used to distract mandibular bone fragments for release of incarcerated soft tissue, and then to reduce the fracture. If more interfragmental compression is needed before fixation is applied, the two **Compression Rolls** are also attached (Reduction-Compression Forceps) to exert uniform compression across the fracture site.

The two sleeves of the compression rolls are secured to the lower border of the mandible with 2.7 mm cortex screws inserted on either side of the fracture, about 1 cm from the fracture line. The tips of the forceps branches are then attached to the threaded ends of the sleeves. After reduction, pressure is exerted across the base of the fracture by tightening the screw lock on the forceps handle, and across the alveolar area by tightening the compression rolls. The reduction compression forceps is also used to effect axial alignment of the fragments in comminuted fractures or in fractures with bone loss (distractor).

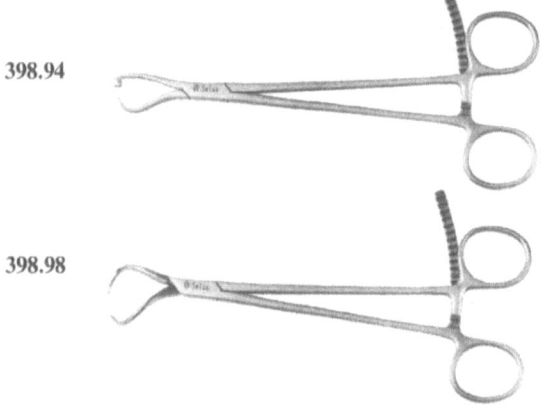

398.94

Holding Forceps for small plates, extra-long

398.98

Reduction Forceps with points, extra-long

for fixation of additional mandibular bone fragments.

399.19
399.49

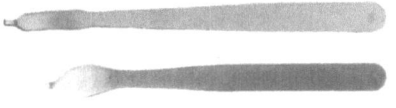
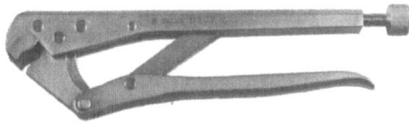

Standard Retractor, 8 mm
Standard Retractor with broad shank

for retracting soft tissues (e.g., during internal fixation in the symphyseal area through an intraoral approach).

329.15

Bending Pliers

for bending mandibular plates. Plate thickness is set with a screw. Plates are bent between holes.

5.4 Supplementary Instruments

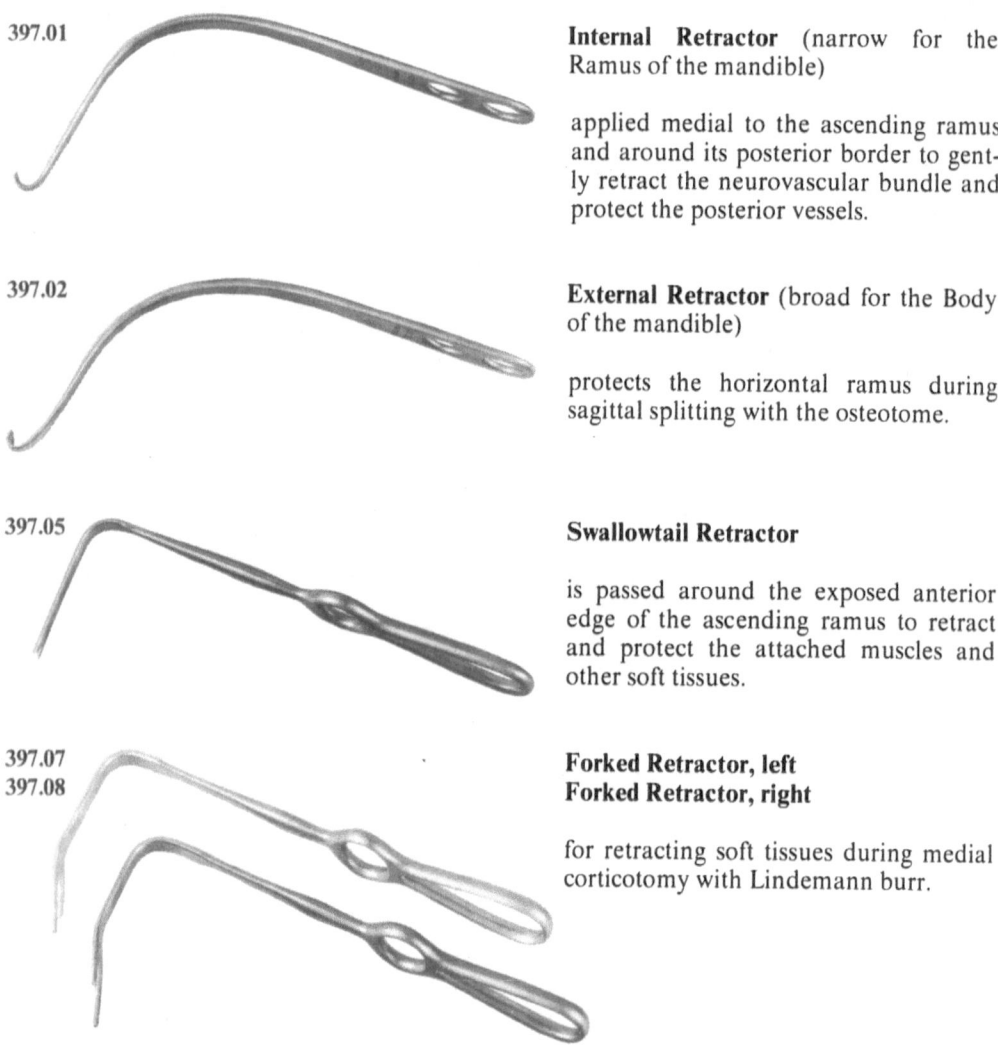

397.01

Internal Retractor (narrow for the Ramus of the mandible)

applied medial to the ascending ramus and around its posterior border to gently retract the neurovascular bundle and protect the posterior vessels.

397.02

External Retractor (broad for the Body of the mandible)

protects the horizontal ramus during sagittal splitting with the osteotome.

397.05

Swallowtail Retractor

is passed around the exposed anterior edge of the ascending ramus to retract and protect the attached muscles and other soft tissues.

397.07
397.08

Forked Retractor, left
Forked Retractor, right

for retracting soft tissues during medial corticotomy with Lindemann burr.

399.80
399.81
399.82

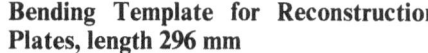

Osteotome, 2 mm, 5 mm and 10 mm

for sagittal split osteotomies.

329.27

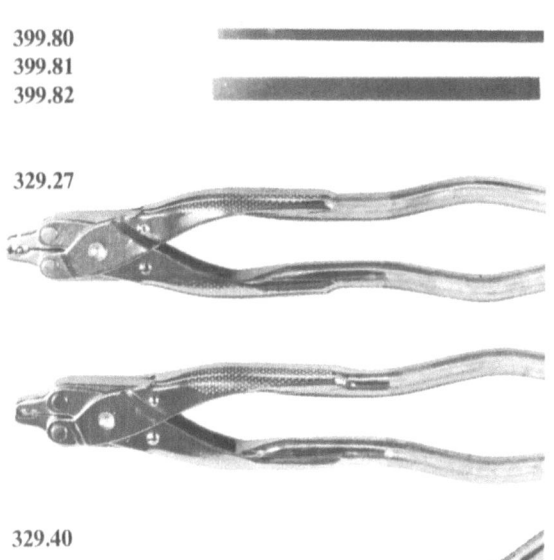

Special Bending Pliers for Reconstruction Plates (2 are required)

for contouring, twisting, and bending along the flat surface or edgewise. Can also be used to shorten reconstruction plates if cutting forceps are not available.

329.40

Bending Template for Reconstruction Plates, length 296 mm

5.5 Cranio Fixateur Externe

The basic equipment of the cranio fixateur externe is the halo with visor and two external and two intraoral fixation elements for stabilization of midfacial fractures. Additional devices are available for intra- and extranasal splinting of the nasal bones and for stabilization of zygomatic and mandibular fractures.

5.5.1 Basic Equipment

395.01

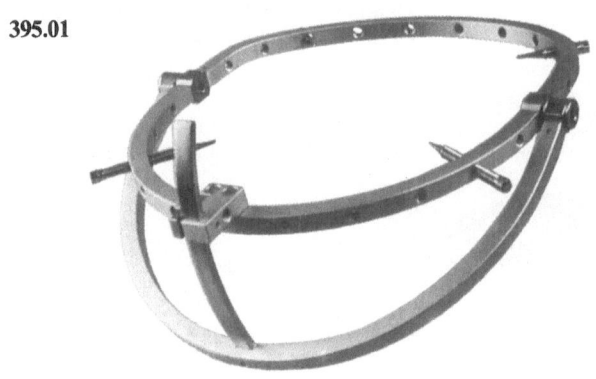

395.02

395.03

395.04

395.30

Halo with visor: The light metal ring with a cranial deviation in the occipital area is anchored in the outer table by six radially oriented **screws (lengths 40, 60, and 85 mm)** using the **6-mm socket wrench.** The screws are placed above the origin of the neck muscles posteriorly and above the hairline anteriorly. The correct orientation of the halo is judged in reference to the midline and the bipupillary line. The visor can be lowered in the frontal plane.

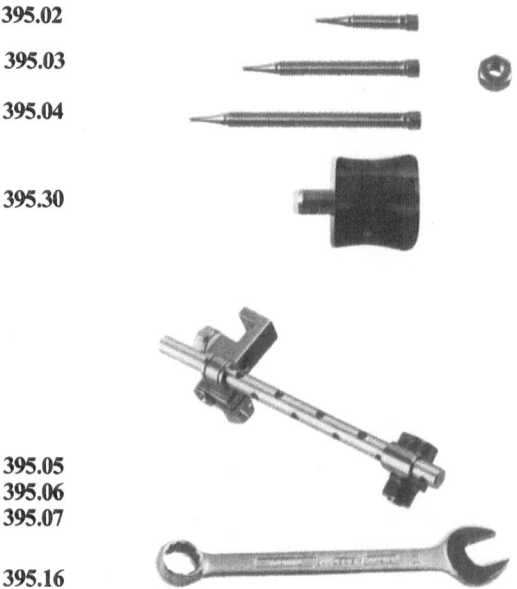

395.05
395.06
395.07

395.16

External fixation elements: parts of a fixateur externe (**suspending clamp, tube,** and **clamp**) as well as additional devices are attached to the visor bilaterally. An **11 mm combination wrench** is necessary.

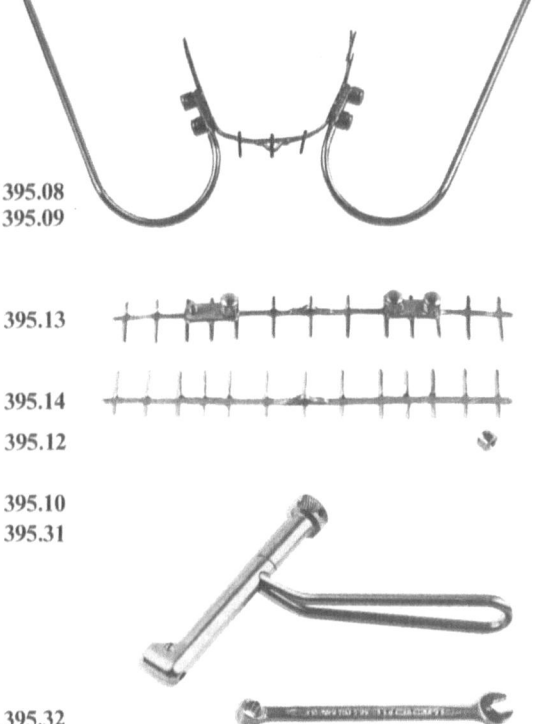

395.08
395.09

395.13

395.14

395.12

395.10
395.31

395.32

The **oral rods** (left and right) connect the external with the intraoral fixation elements.

The intraoral fixation elements comprise the **maxillary arch bar,** which consists of the **arch bar for the mandible** with two incorporated holding plates to which the oral rods can be attached by **nuts.** During application of acryl the holding plates are protected by **rubber protection caps.** For tightening of the nuts the **geared socket wrench** is used as well as a **6 mm combination wrench** (see Fig. 27, p. 34).

5.5.2 Additional Devices

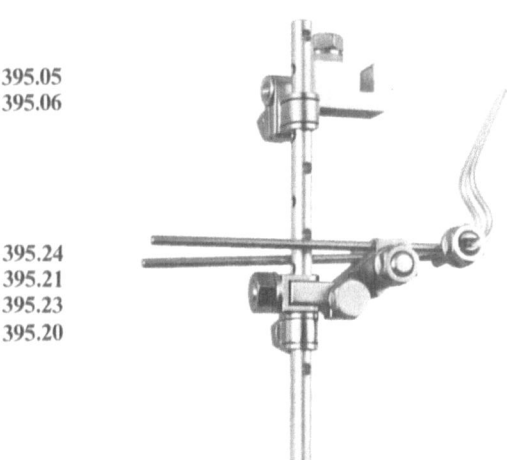

395.05
395.06

395.24
395.21
395.23
395.20

For intranasal splinting a special assembly is used, consisting of the **nasal rods, stop clamp,** and **adjusting screw.**
The **double clamp with hinge,** the **tube** and the **suspending clamp** connect the intranasal assembly with the visor in the midline (see Fig. 29, p. 35).

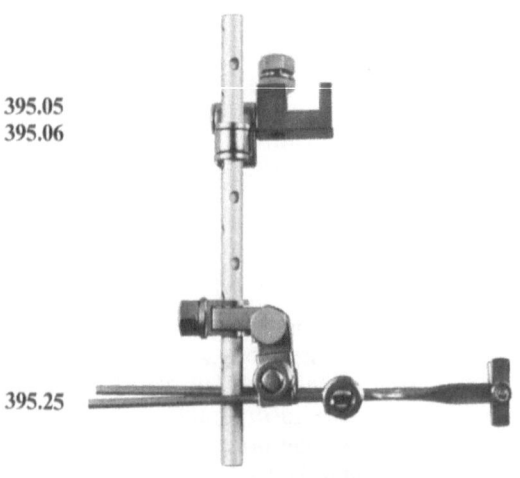

395.05
395.06

395.25

For extranasal splinting, **nasal plates** are used in the place of nasal rods. The rest of the assembly remains as above (see Fig. 30, p. 35).

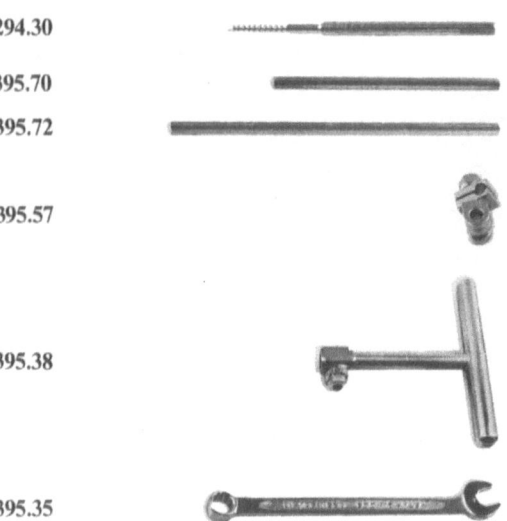

294.30

395.70

395.72

395.57

395.38

395.35

For external fixation of the zygoma, a **Schanz screw** (diameter 4.0 mm, thread diameter 3.5 mm) is inserted and connected to the assembly (395.05-06-07) as previously described (see Fig. 28, p. 34). The stabilization of the mandible is possible with the same Schanz screws connected with **bars** (diameter 4.0 mm, lengths 60 and 100 mm) and **clamps** (diameter 4/4 mm), and, if needed, with the visor.

A simple **handle** is used for inserting the Schanz screws and a **7-mm combination wrench** for tightening the nuts of the clamps.

Note: For details on the cleaning, sterilization and maintenance of instruments, see AO/ASIF Instrumentation, Séquin and Texhammar 1980, p. 219.

6 AO/ASIF Implant Set for Maxillofacial Bone Surgery

102.66*

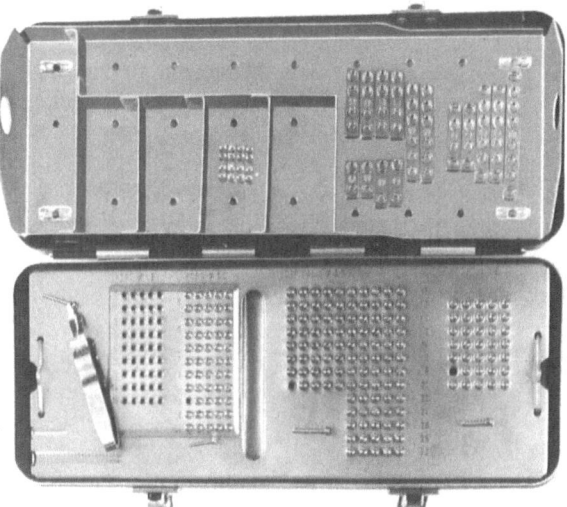

---

* "SYNTHES" Catalogue number

6.1 Screws

201.06–20

2.0 mm Cortex Screws
(flat-spherical head with cruciform recess)

211.06–38

(spherical head with hexagonal socket, width across flats 1.5 mm)

used for fixation of Mini Plates or as lag screws, chiefly in the orbital region.

202.06–32

2.7 mm Cortex Screws
(spherical head with hexagonal socket, width across flats 2.5 mm)

used for fixation of Dynamic Compression Plates (2.7 mm DCP, EDCP, and Reconstruction Plates). Also used as lag screws for sagittal split osteotomies.

203.08–16

Special 3.5 mm screws for mandibular surgery
(5.0 mm dia. spherical head with hexagonal socket, width across flats 2.5 mm)

provide backup in case a 2.7 mm thread is accidentally stripped.

6.2 Plates

243.14

243.16

Mini Plates 2.0
for 2.0 mm Screws with 4 or 6 holes: for plating of the zygoma.

243.09

Adaptionplate
for 2.0 mm screws: can be bent three-dimensionally and cut to desired length.

DCP 2.7
(Dynamic Compression Plates for 2.7 mm Screws)

244.02

244.22

– with 2 holes, small or large center spacing: for tension band plating of the mandibular angle.

244.04

244.06

– with 4 or 6 holes: for infra apical plating in frontal areas, etc.

244.64

244.67

EDCP 2.7
(Mandibular Eccentric Dynamic Compression Plates [outer holes 90° transverse] for 2.7 mm Screws) with 4 or 6 holes.

For use in all fractures that require basal plating of the mandibular border. The plate is attached such that the active edge of the transverse DCP hole is situated basally. The two screws nearest the fracture are inserted first. Then screws are driven in through the transverse holes. With the 6-hole plate, the screws in the intermediate, horizontal holes are the last to be inserted.

Low-eccentricity drilling will produce an effect similar to that of the oblique-hole plate.

Oblique Mandibular Plate for 2.7 mm screws (outer holes 45°)

244.34  – 4 holes, small center spacing

244.35 – 4 holes, large center spacing

244.39 – 5 holes, large center spacing
Function and technique are the same as for the EDCP.

Reconstruction Plates for 2.7 mm screws

These plates are used in the internal fixation of comminuted fractures and fractures with bone loss, and for fixation of the mandibular stumps following osteotomies. They are as narrow as the 2.7 mm DCP and EDCP, but are almost twice as thick. The holes permit dynamic compression to be exerted in both longitudinal directions.

All adjacent plate holes are separated by U-shaped notches which permit the plate to be bent and twisted in any dimension, including edgewise. Contouring is done with the special bending pliers.

245.20–29 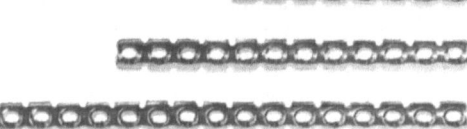 Straight Narrow Reconstruction Plates, 6–24 holes, left and right

245.41–46 Bent Reconstruction Plates

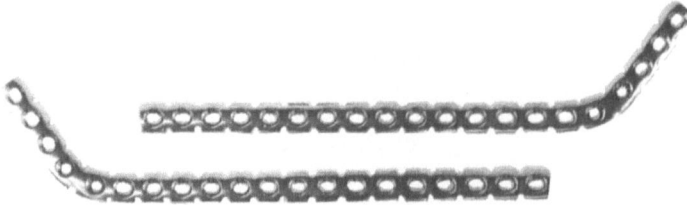

245.51–52

Mandibular Reconstruction Plates

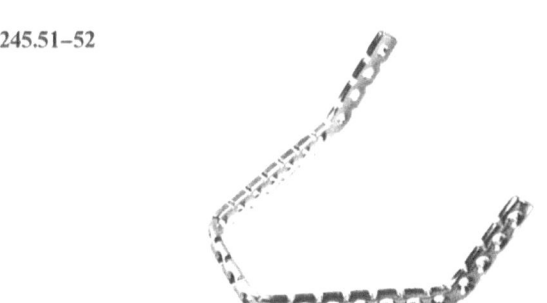

245.61–66

Condylar Prosthesis of the Mandible

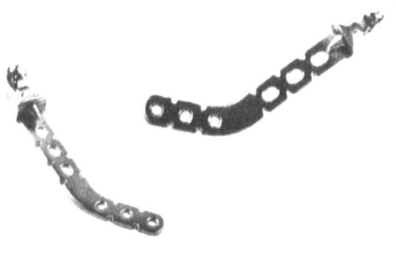

245.71–76

Bent Reconstruction Plates with Condylar Head, left and right

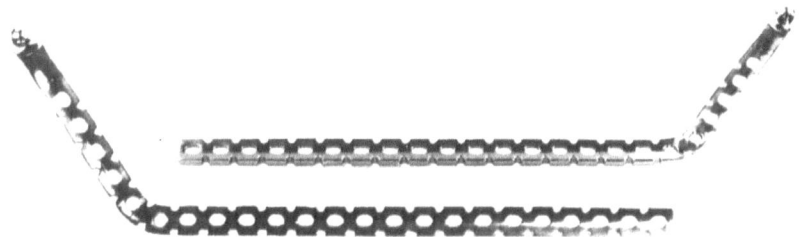

7 AO/ASIF Compressed Air Machines

Compressed air has several advantages as a power source for drilling and cutting machines:

1) Easy availability.

2) Ease of sterilization of compressed air machines.

3) Compressed air machines can be stopped quickly if needed owing to their low inertia. Also, operating speed is easily regulated.

4) Air-powered machines are relatively lightweight.

7.1 Small Air Drill

511.11*

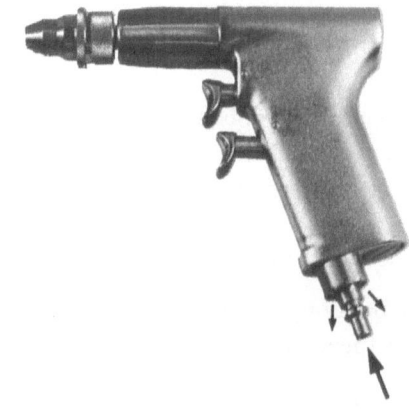

This standard machine is used for drilling holes up to 5 mm in diameter, for tapping, and for the insertion and removal of screws.

Technical Description

- Available in both a single- and double-hose model
- Reversible
- Variable speed up to about 600 rpm
- Quick-coupling chuck for compatible attachments
- Operating pressure: 6 bar (90 psi)
- Air consumption: approx. 250 liters/min
- Weight: approx. 600 g (22 oz)
- Autoclavable to 140 °C (285 °F)

Operation: The speed of the drill is controlled by pressure of the middle finger on the lower trigger. A push on the upper trigger with the index finger reverses the drilling direction (from clockwise to counterclockwise).

Quick Coupling and instruments: Instruments with suitable quick-coupling ends attach to the drill quickly and easily.

Attaching the instruments: Push the sleeve of the coupling forward, insert the end of the instrument into the coupling, and turn it until it engages the keyway. Then insert the end fully and release the sleeve.

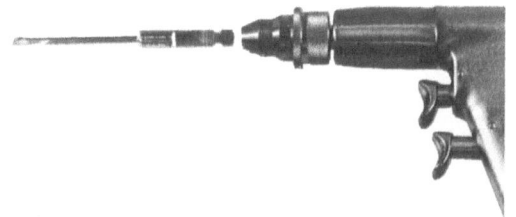

* "SYNTHES" Catalogue number

310.93

310.90

Detaching the instruments: Push the sleeve forward and withdraw the instrument.

A **chuck with key** and **mini quick-coupling chuck** are also available.

Applications:
Drilling: Clockwise operation is normal. Reverse operation is used only occasionally, such as for withdrawing a drill bit.

Necessary Accessories: Pressure-reducing valves, filters, air hoses, oil dispenser, and possibly the lubricating connector, depending on the type of machine and air supply system.

Remarks
- The air supply and exhaust system should be tailored to each operating room.
- Only filtered air supplies should be used.
- Air-operated drills should *never be run on oxygen* due to the danger of fire and explosion.

7.2 Mini Compressed Air Machine and Attachments

112.00

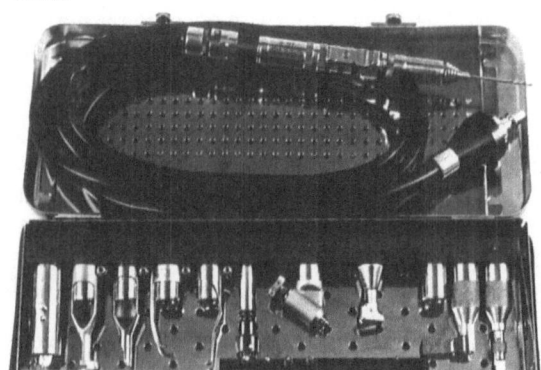

This device was originally developed for hand and mandibular surgery but has proved extremely useful in neurosurgery as well.

The special high-speed machine permits the use of small drill bits and burrs. Special attachments for sawing and chiseling are also available.

Technical Description

- Designed for use with double air hoses only
- Variable speed, 0–15,000 rpm
- Mini quick coupling for compatible instruments
- Operating pressure: 6 bar (90 psi)
- Air consumption: approx. 150 liters/ min
- Weight: approx. 130 g (5 oz.)
- Autoclavable to 140° (285 °F)

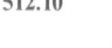
a

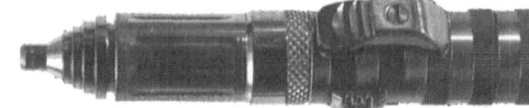

The Air-Driven Motor

permits clockwise operation only. The motor speed is continuously variable from 0–15,000 rpm and is controlled with the large slide switch (*a*).

For greater reliability, a *sterile filter* should always be used to clean the compressed air.

512.15

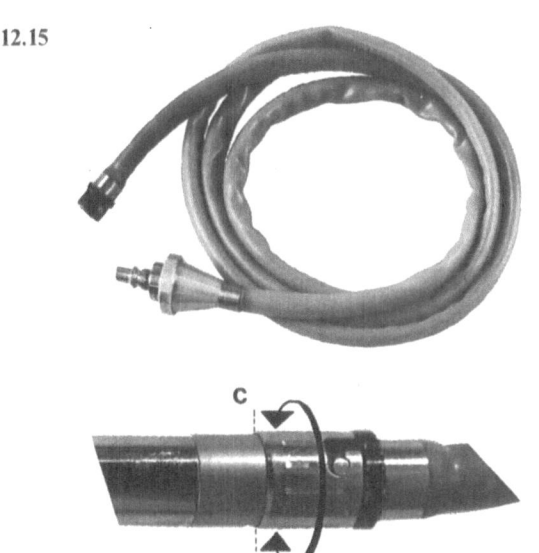

The Double Hose

attaches to the motor by a *swivel coupling* (*a*), which makes the lightweight drill even easier to handle. The exhaust is vented from the operating suite through the outer hose.

The *hose is attached* by grasping the hose coupling (both ends) and inserting it into the coupling of the motor, taking care *not to kink* the hose so that is does not break.

The double-hose nipple fits all standard AO/ASIF double-hose air supply systems.

Attachments (Chucks and Protective Sleeves)

The various *attachments* (chucks, etc.) are connected to the motor by a quick-coupling device. This is done by pushing the small slide (*b*) forward.

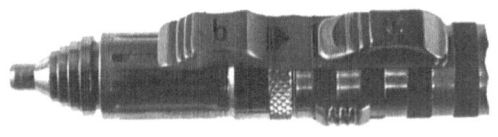

b

512.20

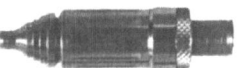

The **straight drill head** has a quick coupling that accepts drill bits and burrs with ends that will fit the standard mini quick coupling.

Instruments are inserted by pulling back the stepped cone, sliding in the instrument shaft, and turning it until the end catches. Then the cone is released.

The standard set contains only drill bits up to 2.7 mm in diameter. If larger holes are required, they can be drilled with a round or straight-edged burr.

The various protective sleeves slip over the cylindrical part of the straight drill head and are held in place with a **small hexagonal screwdriver**.

512.12

512.25 – **Tissue protector for circular saws** up to 15 mm dia.

512.26 – **Tissue protector for burrs** up to 6 mm dia.

512.27 – **Depth stop for drill bits**
(See Synthes catalogue for available drill bits and burrs that are compatible with this drill head.)

512.28 – **Skull guard for trephinations**

512.30 The **90° drill attachment** accepts all drill bits that fit the mini quick coupling. Instruments are inserted by turning the small lever to the right, sliding the instrument in, and turning it until the end catches. The small lever is then turned back to lock the instrument in place.

512.40 The **45° drill attachment** has a cannulated chuck for Kirschner wires of 0.6–2.0 mm dia. (0.8–1.7 mm in older models). Pressing on the small lever (*f*) until it clicks into place will lock the gears while the chuck is being tightened to secure the Kirschner wire.
The built-in reduction gears reduce the drill speed to a maximum of 4500 rpm.

512.70

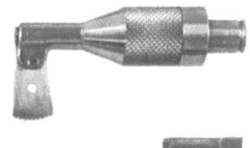

The **oscillating saw** attachment is used for the high-precision sawing of bone.

512.75
512.76

The **saw blade** is attached by slipping it over the mushroom-shaped guide parallel to the machine axis, then turning it 90° into the operating position (it must slip into the slot of the plunger). It is locked on the carrier bolt by pressing upward.
The blade is removed by reversing these steps.
The teeth of the saw blades have a special set, and so they cannot be resharpened. Worn blades are discarded.

512.50

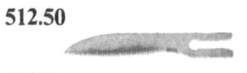

512.55

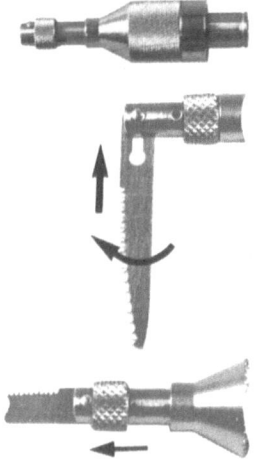

Reciprocating Saw

The **saw blade** is attached by inserting it into the slot at right angles to the machine axis. After the blade is rotated about the carrier pin, it can be locked in place with the retaining ring.
The blade is removed by reversing these steps.

References

Allgöwer M (1969) A dynamic compression plate. Acta Orthop Scand 125:29

Allgöwer M (1975) Grundsätzliches zur Osteosynthese. Fortschr Kiefer Gesichtschir 19:1

Allgöwer M, Perren SM, Matter P (1970) A new plate for internal fixation – The Dynamic Compression Plate (DCP). Injury 2:40

Allgöwer M, Kinzl L, Matter P, Perren SM, Rüedi T (1973) Die dynamische Kompressionsplatte DCP. Springer, Berlin Heidelberg New York

Bronz G, Schmoker R, Tschopp H (1983) Le fratture della mandibola: analisi di 127 casi. Gaz Med Tic 4:169

Claudi B, Spiessl B (1975) Ergebnisse bei konservativer und operativer Behandlung von Unterkieferfrakturen (ohne Collumfrakturen). Fortschr Kiefer Gesichtschir 19:73

Eschmann A (1975) Ergebnisse der Nachuntersuchungen bei 101 Patienten mit funktionsstabiler Unterkieferosteosynthese. Med. Dissertation, Universität Basel

Galeazzi G (1972) Experimentelle Untersuchungen zur intraoperativen Druckveränderung bei der Plattenosteosynthese. Med. Dissertation, Universität Basel

Ganz R, Perren SM, Rueter A (1975) Mechanische Induktion der Knochenresorption. Fortschr Kiefer Gesichtschir 19:45

Gebauer U (1977) Elektronische Meß- und Rechenanlage zur arcogrammetrischen Modelldiagnostik und zum Auswerten von Fernröntgenbildern. Schweiz Monatsschr Zahnheilkd 87:1170

Jaques WA (1976) Preventive antiobiotics in elective maxillofacial surgery. In: Spiessl B (ed) New concepts in maxillofacial bone surgery. Springer, Berlin Heidelberg New York, p 175

Krüger E (1974) Die operative Behandlung des offenen Bisses durch dreiteilende Osteotomie des Oberkiefers. Fortschr Kiefer Gesichtschir 18:211

Martinoni G, Tschopp H (1976) The surgical approach in the treatment of facial fractures. In: Spiessl B (ed) New concepts in maxillofacial bone surgery. Springer, Berlin Heidelberg New York, p 75

Matter P, Brennwald J, Perren SM (1974) Biologische Reaktion des Knochens auf Osteosyntheseplatten. Helv Chir Acta Suppl. 12

Müller ME, Allgöwer M, Schneider R, Willenegger H (1977) Manual der Osteosynthese. Springer, Berlin Heidelberg New York

Niederdellmann H (1975) Elektronische Messungen zur Biomechanik bei Osteosynthesen im Unterkiefer. Fortschr Kiefer Gesichtschir 19:42

Niederdellmann H, Schilli WG (1972) Funktionsstabile Osteosynthese im Unterkiefer. Dtsch Zahnärztl Z 27:138

Obwegeser HL, Sailer HF (1978) Experiences with intraoral partial resection and simultaneous reconstruction in cases of mandibular osteomyelitis. J Maxillofac Surg 6:34

Perren SM, Rahn B, Cordey J (1975) Mechanik und Biologie der Frakturheilung. Fortschr Kiefer Gesichtschir 19:33

Prein J, Eschmann A, Spiessl B (1976) Ergebnisse der Nachuntersuchung bei 81 Patienten mit funktionsstabiler Unterkieferosteosynthese. Fortschr Kiefer Gesichtschir 21:304

Prein J, Spiessl B, Rahn B, Perren SM (1975) Frakturheilung am Unterkiefer nach operativer Versorgung. Eine tierexperimentelle Studie. Fortschr Kiefer Gesichtschir 19:17

Rahn B (1976) Die polychrome Sequenzmarkierung. Habilitationsschrift, Universität Freiburg

Rahn B, Cordey J, Prein J, Russenberger M (1975) Zur Biomechanik der Osteosynthese an der Mandibula. Fortschr Kiefer Gesichtschir 19:37

Rittmann WW, Perren SM (1974) Corticale Knochenheilung nach Osteosynthese und Infektion. Springer, Berlin Heidelberg New York

Rittmann WW, Matter P, Brennwald J, Kayer F, Perren SM (1975) Biologie und Biomechanik infizierter Osteosynthesen. Fortschr Kiefer Gesichtschir 19:48

Rüedi T (1972) und AO-Bulletin (1975/1976) Zur Behandlung der posttraumatischen Osteomyelitis. Zentralbl Chir 97:1634

Sailer HF (1976) Ergebnisse der gleichzeitigen Resektion und Rekonstruktion des Unterkiefers auf oralem Wege. Fortschr Kiefer Gesichtschir 20:45

Schenk R (1975) Histologie der primären Knochenheilung. Fortschr Kiefer Gesichtschir 19:8

Schilli W, Niederdellmann H (1980) Verletzungen des Gesichtsschädels. Huber, Bern

Schmoker R (1973) Exzentrisch dynamische Kompressionsplatte sowie Kompressions-Zuggurtungsschiene, Kompressions-Zuggurtungsplatte und Repositions-Kompressionszange. Eine neue Technik der funktionsstabilen Unterkieferosteosynthese mit Kompression auf der Zugseite. Med. Dissertation, Universität Basel

Schmoker R (1975a) Experimentelle Untersuchungen zur Stabilität und intraoperativen Kompressionserzeugung von Osteosynthesen bei Unterkieferfrakturen. AO-Bulletin, Bern

Schmoker R (1975b) Zur Operationsplanung bei Progenie- und Retrogeniefällen. Schweiz Monatsschr Zahnheilkd 85:598

Schmoker R (1976a) The eccentric dynamic compression plate. An experimental study as to it's contribution to the functionally stable internal fixation of fractures of the lower jaw. AO-Bulletin, Bern

Schmoker R (1976b) Internal fixation of mandibular fractures using an eccentric dynamic compression plate (EDCP). In: Spiessl B (ed) New concepts in maxillofacial bone surgery. Springer, Berlin Heidelberg New York

Schmoker R (1982) Rigid internal fixation of compound fractures of the mandible using a specially designed reconstruction plate. International symposium on Maxillofacial Trauma, Nov 13–15 Detroit, Michigan. Jacobs, Maxillofacial Trauma. Praeger, in press

Schmoker R (1983a) Der Craniofixateur externe zur funktionsstabilen Fixation des Mittelgesichts. Erfahrungsbericht nach Anwendung in über 50 Fällen. Dtsch Z Mund Kiefer Gesichtschir 7:235

Schmoker R (1983b) Mandibular reconstruction using a special plate. Animal experiments and clinical application. J Maxillofac Surg 11:99

Schmoker R, Gebauer U (1980) Präoperative Planung und funktionsstabile Fixation mittels Osteosynthesen und Craniofixateur externe bei der Behandlung der Progenie, des offenen Bisses sowie des Distalbisses. Schweiz Monatsschr Zahnheilkd 90:286

Schmoker R, Spiessl B (1973) Exzentrisch dynamische Kompressionsplatte. Schweiz Monatsschr Zahnheilkd 83:12

Schmoker R, Spiessl B (1976) Infektion nach Osteosynthese von Unterkieferfrakturen. Kasuistik, Ursache, Verhütung, Behandlung. Aktuel Traumatol 6:297

Schmoker R, Spiessl B (1978) Fehlermöglichkeiten bei der Osteosynthese von Unterkieferfrakturen. Dtsch Z Mund Kiefer Gesichtschir 2:129

Schmoker R, Spiessl B (1979) Umstellungsosteotomie des Oberkiefers und Ruhigstellung mittels Craniofixateur. Schweiz Monatsschr Zahnheilkd 89:287

84

Schmoker R, Tschopp HM (1979a) Präoperative Planung der sagittalen Spaltungs-osteotomie mittels Simulographie. Dtsch Z Mund Kiefer Gesichtschir 3:37

Schmoker R, Tschopp HM (1979b) Prinzipien zur Versorgung von Gesichtsfraktu-ren. Helv Chir Acta 46:39

Schmoker R, Spiessl B, Holtgrave E, Schotland C (1975) Ergebnisse der operativen Versorgung von Jochbeinfrakturen. Fortschr Kiefer Gesichtschir 19:154

Schmoker R, Spiessl B, Mathys R (1976a) A total mandibular plate to bridge large defects of the mandible. In: Spiessl B (ed) New concepts in maxillofacial bone surgery. Springer, Berlin Heidelberg New York

Schmoker R, Spiessl B, Tschopp HM, Prein J, Jacques WA (1976b) Die funktions-stabile Osteosynthese am Unterkiefer mittels exzentrisch dynamischer Kompres-sionsplatte (EDCP). Ergebnisse einer Nachuntersuchung der ersten 25 Fälle. Schweiz Monatsschr Zahnheilkd 86:167

Schmoker R, Spiessl B, Mathys R (1977a) Eine Rekonstruktionsplatte zur Über-brückung größerer Knochendefekte im Unterkiefer. Aktuel Traumatol 7:199

Schmoker R, Eulenberger J, Spiessl B, Mathys R (1977b) Entwicklung und tierexpe-rimentelle Untersuchung einer Kieferköpfchenprothese. Dtsch Z Mund Kiefer Gesichtschir 1:86

Schmoker R, Spiessl B, Dillier R (1979) Operative Behandlung des offenen Bisses und der alveolären Protrusion. Fortschr Kieferorthop 40:61

Schmoker R, Allmen G von, Tschopp HM (1981) Der künstliche Ersatz des Kiefer-gelenks. Schweiz Monatsschr Zahnheilkd 31:222

Schmoker R, Allmen G von, Tschopp HM (1982) Application of Functionally Stable Fixation in Maxillofacial Surgery according to the ASIF Principles. J Oral Surg 40:457

Séquin F, Texhammar R (1980) Das AO-Instrumentarium. Springer Berlin Heidel-berg New York

Séquin F, Texhammar R (1981) AO/ASIF Instrumentation. Springer, Berlin Heidel-berg New York

Spiessl B (1971) Scope of orthodontic treatment in adults combined with oral surgery. Trans Europ Orthodont Soc

Spiessl B (1974) Osteosynthese bei sagittaler Osteotomie nach OBWEGESER/DAL PONT. Fortschr Kiefer Gesichtschir 18:145

Spiessl B (1975) Die funktionsstabile Osteosynthese bei Unterkieferfrakturen. Pro-blematik, Indikation und Technik. Fortschr Kiefer Gesichtschir 19:68

Spiessl B (1976a) Grundsätzliches zur Knochentransplantation. Fortschr Kiefer Ge-sichtschir 20:14

Spiessl B (1976b) New concepts in maxillofacial bone surgery. Springer, Berlin Hei-delberg New York

Spiessl B (1976c) Rigid internal fixation after sagittal split osteotomy of the ascend-ing ramus. In: Spiessl B (ed) New concepts in maxillofacial bone surgery. Sprin-ger, Berlin Heidelberg New York, p 115

Spiessl B (1981) A new method of anatomical reconstruction of extensive defects of the mandible with autogenous cancellous bone. J Maxillofac Surg 8:78

Spiessl B, Schargus G (1971) Planung prä- und postoperativer Behandlung bei kie-ferorthopädischen Eingriffen. Dtsch Z Stomatol 21:734

Spiessl B, Schroll K (1972) Gesichtsschädel. In: Nigst H (Hrsg) Spezielle Frakturen-und Luxationslehre. Thieme, Stuttgart

Spiessl B, Tschopp HM (1974) Orthopädische Operationen am Kiefer. In: Naumann H (Hrsg) Gesicht und Gesichtsschädel. Thieme, Stuttgart

Spiessl B, Schargus G, Schroll K (1971) Die stabile Osteosynthese bei Frakturen des unbezahnten Unterkiefers. Schweiz Monatsschr Zahnheilk 81:39

Spiessl B, Schmoker R, Mathys R (1976a) Treatment of an ankylosis by a condylar prosthesis of the mandible. In: Spiessl B (ed) New concepts in maxillofacial bone surgery. Springer, Berlin Heidelberg New York, p 83

Spiessl B, Prein J, Schmoker R (1976 b) Anatomical reconstruction and functional rehabilitation of mandibular defects after ablative surgery. In: Spiessl B (ed) New concepts in maxillofacial bone surgery. Springer, Berlin Heidelberg New York, p 160

Tschopp H (1976) Clinical aspects of free autogenous bone transplantation. Spiessl B (ed) New concepts in maxillofacial bone surgery. Springer, Berlin Heidelberg New York, p 3

Tschopp H, Martinoni G (1976) Principles in treatment in combined fractures of the upper and lower jaw. In: Spiessl B (ed) New concepts in maxillofacial bone surgery. Springer, Berlin Heidelberg New York, p 63

Subject Index

New Concepts in Maxillofacial Bone Surgery

Editor: **B. Spiessl**

With contributions by C. Bassetti, D. Cornoley, T. Gensheimer, H. Graf, E. Holtgrave, W. Huser, W.-A. Jaques, G. Martinoni, R. Mathys, J. Prein, T. Rakosi, W. Remagen, R. Schmoker, B. Spiessl, H.M. Tschopp

1976. 183 figures, 36 tables. XIII, 194 pages. ISBN 3-540-07929-7

Contents: Transplantation of Autogenous Bone. – Traumatology and Reconstructive Surgery. – Orthopaedic Maxillofacial Surgery. – Implantology. – Postoperative Infections and Prophylaxis. – References. – Subject Index.

"This book deals with numerous aspects of maxillofacial bone surgery, with special emphasis on the stability of fixation in fracture treatment and osteotomies. The compression plate-osteosynthesis is dealt with in detail. Fifteen authors have contributed to this excellent book. Many chapters deserve special comment: transplantation of autogeneous bone, traumatology and reconstructive surgery, orthopedic maxillofacial surgery, implantology and postoperative infections and prophylaxis. The book is, as other Springer publications, elegantly presented, with excellent reproduction of radiographs and numerous instructive drawings."

International Journal of Oral Surgery

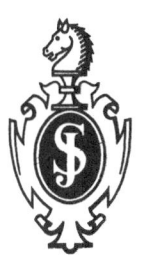

Springer-Verlag
Berlin
Heidelberg
New York
Tokyo

F. Sequin, R. Texhammar

AO/ASIF Instrumentation

Manual of Use and Care

Introduction and Scientific Aspects by H. Willenegger
Translated from the German by T. Telger
1981. Approx. 1300 figures, 17 separated checklists.
XVI, 306 pages. ISBN 3-540-10337-6

Contents: Introduction. – Medical and Scientific
Directives. – Principles of the AO/ASIF-Technique
and Basic Mechanical Principles. – Practical Part:
Instrumentation of the AO/ASIF. Compressed Air
and Compressed-Air Machines. Cleaning, Care, and
Sterilization of Instruments and Implants. Preoperative, Operative, and Postoperative Guidelines. Suggestions for the Management of Various Fractures.
Preparation of the Instruments. – Subject Index.

Manual of Internal Fixation

Techniques Recommended by the AO Group

By **M.E. Müller, M. Allgöwer, R. Schneider,
H. Willenegger**

In collaboration with W. Bandi, A. Boitzy, R. Ganz,
U. Heim, S.M. Perren, W.W. Rittmann, T. Rüedi,
B.G. Weber, S. Weller
Translated from the German by J. Schatzker
2nd, expanded and revised edition. 1979. 345 figures,
2 Templates for Preoperative Planning. X, 409 pages.
ISBN 3-540-09227-7

Contents: Introduction. – General Considerations:
Aims and Fundamental Principles of the AO Method.
Means by Which Stable Internal Fixation is Achieved.
Preoperative, Operative und Postoperative Guidelines. – Special Part: Internal Fixation of Fresh Fractures: Closed Fractures in the Adult. Open Fractures
in the Adult. Fractures in Children. – Supplement:
Reconstructive Bone Surgery. Delayed Union. Pseudarthroses. Osteotomies. Arthrodeses. – Bibliography.
– Index.

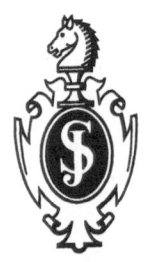

Springer-Verlag
Berlin
Heidelberg
New York
Tokyo